CLEAN
PALEO
COMFORT
FOOD
Cookbook

For Joanna.

You bring me more joy than I ever knew possible.

————

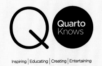

Brimming with creative inspiration, how-to projects, and useful information to enrich your everyday life, Quarto Knows is a favorite destination for those pursuing their interests and passions. Visit our site and dig deeper with our books into your area of interest: Quarto Creates, Quarto Cooks, Quarto Homes, Quarto Lives, Quarto Drives, Quarto Explores, Quarto Gifts, or Quarto Kids.

First Published in 2021 by Fair Winds Press, an imprint of The Quarto Group, 100 Cummings Center, Suite 265-D, Beverly, MA 01915, USA.
T (978) 282-9590 F (978) 283-2742 QuartoKnows.com

Fair Winds Press titles are also available at discount for retail, wholesale, promotional, and bulk purchase. For details, contact the Special Sales Manager by email at specialsales@quarto.com or by mail at The Quarto Group, Attn: Special Sales Manager, 100 Cummings Center, Suite 265-D, Beverly, MA 01915, USA.

25 24 23 22 21   1 2 3 4 5

ISBN: 978-1-59233-985-3

Digital edition published in 2021

Library of Congress Cataloging-in-Publication Data

Names: DeMay, Jessica, author.
Title: Clean paleo comfort food cookbook : 100 delicious recipes that nourish body & soul / Jessica DeMay.
Description: Beverly, MA : Fair Winds Press, 2021. | Includes index. |
Identifiers: LCCN 2020030167 (print) | LCCN 2020030168 (ebook) | ISBN 9781592339853 (trade paperback) | ISBN 9781631599675 (ebook)
Subjects: LCSH: Gluten-free diet--Recipes. | Gluten-free foods. | Comfort food. | Prehistoric peoples--Food. | LCGFT: Cookbooks.
Classification: LCC RM237.86 .D44 2021 (print) | LCC RM237.86 (ebook) |
    DDC 641.5/639311--dc23

Design: Allison Meierding
Page Layout: Allison Meierding
Food Photography: Joe St.Pierre Photography
             @joestpierre
Lifestyle Photography: Emily DeKoster Photography
Food Styling: Joy Howard | joyfoodstyle.com

Printed in China

————

The information in this book is for educational purposes only. It is not intended to replace the advice of a physician or medical practitioner. Please see your health-care provider before beginning any new health program.

CLEAN PALEO COMFORT FOOD

Cookbook

100 Delicious Recipes That Nourish Body & Soul

Jessica DeMay

FAIR WINDS

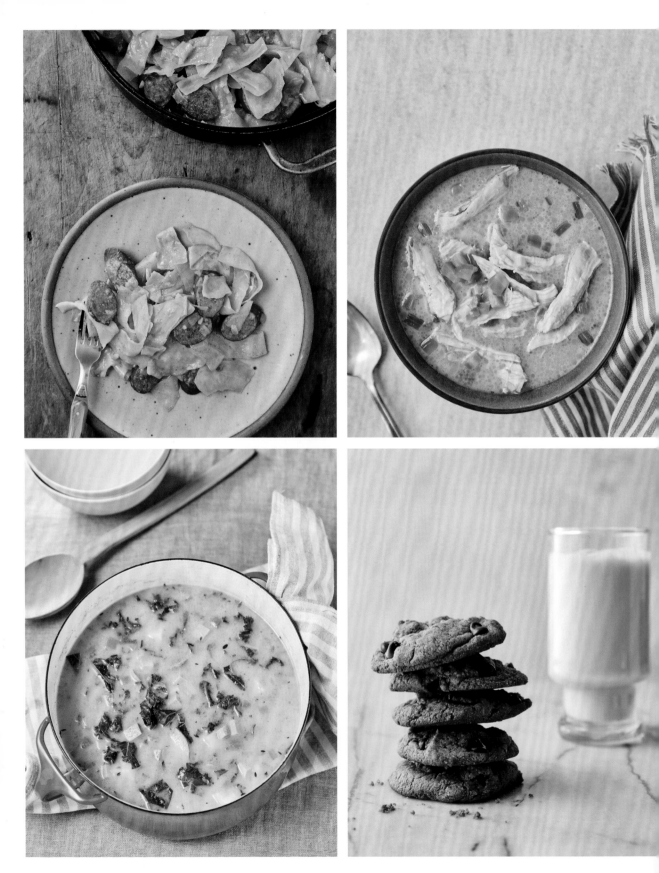

contents

my story

My health struggles began with thyroid issues when I was a teenager—I found myself dealing with fatigue, heavy periods, and an enlarged thyroid gland. I was diagnosed with and put on medicine for hypothyroidism. The medicine I was on pushed me into hyper-thyroidism, giving me late-stage osteoporosis when I was just seventeen years old. My doctor gave me radioactive iodine to destroy my thy-roid, so it didn't weaken my bones further. I will be on thyroid medicine for the rest of my life.

Then, for seven years, from age nineteen to twenty-six, I struggled with an eating disorder that almost took my life. I was hospitalized multiple times, became too sick to work, and dropped to a very low weight. The last time I was hospitalized, during the fall of 2013, I went into a coma for a few days. It scared me to think I could have died from the choices I had been making. It made me realize how serious it was, and it was my wake-up call to get healthy.

I started to care about nourishing my body. I was gaining weight, and I wanted to do so in a healthy way. I'm thirty-three now and the healthiest I have ever been: I'm at a healthy weight, and I have a great relationship with food. And paleo has helped me get here. Even though it can be seen as restrictive, it has actually been the opposite for me, giving me confidence to eat more fat and calories than I ever have. I still enjoy treats, eggs (not just the whites!), snacks, and, of course, full meals. It was worth it to me to feel so much better. To anyone who has struggled with an eating disorder or been obsessive over food, I encourage you not to count calories. Trust your body as you are feeding it nourishing food.

After recovery from my eating disorder, I still dealt with some physical symptoms that I didn't think were a big deal, but definitely weren't normal for my age. I was in my twenties and had arthritis in my knees and breakouts on my face. I knew this was common and didn't worry about it much. Once I completely gave up grains and dairy, my knee pain went away and my face cleared up.

Back when I was a teenager, food had never even been considered as an option for treating my thyroid issues. But perhaps food choices could have helped with my issues. Since I switched to a paleo lifestyle, my bone density has improved. I have been able to stay off prescription drugs to increase my bone den-sity; I've worked on bone strength naturally by taking collagen and vitamin D and doing weight-bearing exercise a few times a week.

I was not raised in a household in which my mom or grandma taught me how to cook. I don't have those memories, but that doesn't mean my passion for food is any less. I am a self-taught cook, and I learned to bake before I learned to cook. I got into baking as a teenager and found a deep love for it. Starting with plain ingredients and turning them into a delicious treat was a way for me to unwind and relieve stress. I even won some baking competitions, which gave me enough courage to start my blog, *Real Food with Jessica*. Paleo baking is different, of course, and there's a learning curve, but it's incredibly rewarding. I love that I can bake and share these recipes with people who are missing treats.

Note: This is my personal story. I am not a doctor or dietitian; I'm just sharing what has worked for me. Consult your doctor for a plan that works for you.

How to Use This Book

All the recipes in this book are easy enough for a cook with any level of experience to make. Some are quicker and have shorter ingredient lists than others, but none are overly complicated. I love recipes with short ingredient lists and quick steps, but I won't sacrifice flavor for ease. Sometimes it's worth it to take the time to make the more involved dishes. I like to save those for the weekend, when time isn't as pressed.

Be sure to read every recipe through entirely before starting. This will help ensure you are making it correctly and adding ingredients at the right time.

There is a chapter of basics that are easy to make, but most of these are now available as store-bought items. Don't feel like every ingredient needs to be homemade to make it a successful dish. Take shortcuts where needed to make a recipe work for you. It's more affordable to make condiments from scratch, but it's less time-consuming to buy paleo versions in the store. Both are equally good options.

Each recipe has a key labeling it nut free, egg free, and/or low FODMAP, when appropriate, so you can tell right away whether it fits your needs.

I love getting my daughter involved in the kitchen; even at a young age, she can add ingredients to a bowl, stir, and scoop. She has a kid's knife to help cut fruit and veggies, and we have a good time together. She is always more likely to try a food she helped prepare as well, which is an added benefit.

I would love for you to find a friend, child, or significant other with whom to share the cooking experience. It is more fun and rewarding when you're cooking, eating, and even cleaning up with someone. You are creating positive memories and an enjoyable experience around food. Enjoy!

Jessica

Chapter 1

comfort food paleo

Comfort food paleo is all about taking real ingredients and creating something that is hearty, nostalgic, and enjoyable.

When I started my food blog in 2015, people responded well to the comfort food dishes I was making. They loved the healthier takes on the Sloppy Joes, casseroles, and baked goods that they were familiar with. And they inspired this book! I have recreated some of our favorite familiar flavors and dishes so you can continue to enjoy them. The dishes I create are inspired by meals I grew up eating or cooked before transitioning to a paleo lifestyle. They're remade to be grain free and dairy free. My hope is that you'll continue making memories around the new versions of these dishes. After all, completely giving up your favorite foods isn't sustainable, but recreating them is! Eating paleo definitely doesn't have to mean salads for every meal or plain chicken breast. It can mean exciting food the whole family will enjoy.

I am not claiming these recipes are low calorie or low fat, because that is not the point of paleo. The focus should be on eating nourishing foods and not worrying about calorie counts. I don't like it when recipes are labeled "guilt-free" or "skinny." Food should never make you feel guilty. It may make you physically feel unwell, which is why you choose to not consume it, but you shouldn't feel shame over what you eat. I don't create recipes to be guilt-free, but free from ingredients that may not work well with your body. My recipes fall in a wide range of low-carb, low-fat to high-carb or high-fat dishes. They are all, however, made with whole food ingredients that will nourish your body and make you feel satisfied.

What Is Paleo?

Paleo is a diet or lifestyle that eliminates certain foods that can be inflammatory or irritating to our digestive system. It focuses on real, nutrient-dense food. Getting grass-fed beef, pasture-raised chicken and pork, pasture-raised eggs, and wild-caught seafood is very important. Not only are they healthier options, but they are also more humane for the animal while they're alive, and that matters so much. Paleo has a reputation for being heavy on meat and bacon, but it's much more balanced than that. Try to fill your plate with vegetables at every meal. Let meat be a part of that, but not the main part. Also, carbs are definitely allowed. Sweet potatoes, plantains, white potatoes, and winter squash are some examples of carb sources, and there is no set amount to have or avoid. Every body is different. The amount you need depends on your fitness and health condition.

When paleo first became popular, it was viewed as the caveman diet, modeled after what cavemen ate. I don't think that is the best representation, because cavemen didn't bake desserts or have pans to cook with. I think a better emphasis is just a focus on real food—eating foods in their most natural state, fresh when possible, and not focusing on calorie counting.

Paleo is also known for going deeper into the source of food—buying the most humane possible version that fits in the budget and thinking about sustainability. After I switched to a paleo lifestyle, I started caring and learning about the source of my food. We'll talk about this more when we discuss reading labels on the packages of meat and eggs. But do also pay attention to the foods you buy from other countries, such as cacao, coconut (oil, flour), and coffee. Buying fair trade means the farmers who grew your food were paid a livable wage and have safe working conditions. I know everyone is at a different point in their journey, but I hope you learn a little bit more about animal and human treatment and consider paying a little extra for those products. It really makes a difference.

Paleo versus Clean Paleo

Some people reintroduce certain food groups into their diets after eating paleo for a certain period. Sometimes they follow the 80/20 rule, meaning they follow a strict paleo diet 80 percent of the time and eat non-paleo food the other 20 percent of the time. This is not the approach of this book. All recipes in this book are 100 percent paleo and have no reintroductions. Every ingredient is totally paleo-compliant with no substitutions needed.

Which Foods to Eat

Here's an overview of which foods are considered paleo, but it's so important to listen to your body and decide whether a certain food works well for you or not. I know a lot of people have egg sensitivities, so even though eggs are paleo, eggs don't work for them. That is really the goal of eating paleo: to find the foods that make you feel your best and eliminate the ones that make you feel terrible.

MEATS

Always try to get the best you can afford. Grass-fed beef is ideal. Grass-fed is even more important than organic because grass-fed meat is more likely to be free of hormones and antibiotics, has up to five times more omega-3s than factory-farmed meat, and is higher in vitamins A and E. Pasture-raised chicken is better than conventional because it contains more omega-3 fats and has more vitamin A. Pasture-raised pork is the best option because it's higher in selenium (an antioxidant) and vitamin E. Pasture-raised eggs are the preferred choice because they contain more vitamin E, omega-3 fats, and beta-carotene. Buying pasture-raised and grass-fed meat and pasture-raised eggs is also about animal welfare. Those animals have been treated humanely, having been given room to roam rather than kept in a cage or barn their whole life.

- Beef
- Bison
- Chicken
- Clams
- Eggs
- Lobster
- Pork
- Wild-caught fish
- Wild game: venison, rabbit, elk

VEGETABLES AND FRUIT

Almost all fruits and vegetables are allowed, except for corn and peas. Corn is so genetically modified that it is considered a grain, and peas are technically a legume. Buying all organic can be expensive, so I suggest using the Clean Fifteen and Dirty Dozen lists. These lists are put out every year by the Environmental Working Group (EWG), and they show the produce with the highest and lowest levels of pesticides (see ewg.org/foodnews for the most up-to-date lists). I always buy organic for something on the Dirty Dozen list, but I won't always if it's on the Clean Fifteen.

> **Clean Fifteen 2020**: Avocados, corn (not paleo), pineapples, sweet peas frozen (not paleo), onions, papayas, eggplants, asparagus, kiwis, cabbage, cauliflower, cantaloupe, broccoli, mushrooms, honeydew.
>
> **Dirty "Dozen" 2020**: Strawberries, spinach, kale, nectarines, apples, grapes, peaches, cherries, pears, tomatoes, celery, potatoes, hot peppers.

- Acorn squash
- Apples
- Apricots
- Arugula
- Asparagus
- Avocados
- Bananas
- Bell peppers
- Berries (strawberries, blueberries, raspberries, cherries, blackberries)
- Broccoli
- Butternut squash
- Carrots
- Cauliflower
- Celery
- Cherries
- Coconut
- Cucumbers
- Eggplant
- Grapefruit
- Grapes
- Green beans
- Green onions
- Kale
- Kiwi
- Lemons
- Lettuce (butter, iceberg, romaine)
- Limes
- Mushrooms
- Onions
- Oranges
- Papayas
- Peaches
- Pears
- Plantains
- Pomegranates
- Spaghetti squash
- Spinach
- Sweet potatoes
- Tomatoes
- Watermelon
- White potatoes
- Zucchini

NUTS AND SEEDS

Nuts and seeds are a great source of healthy fats and protein. Be sure to check that there are no unhealthy oils added to the nuts. Peanut and canola oil are often added, and you want to avoid them. Buying raw or dry-roasted nuts is always a good choice. Remember that peanuts are not allowed, as they are actually a legume. Also, if you can afford it or want to try it yourself, sprouting the nuts makes them easier to digest and helps your body absorb the nutrients better.

- Almonds
- Brazil nuts
- Cashews
- Hazelnuts
- Macadamias
- Pecans
- Pine nuts
- Pumpkin seeds
- Sesame seeds
- Sunflower seeds
- Walnuts

HEALTHY FATS

Fat has gotten a bad reputation for years. It is great for your body, fills you up, and is a good energy source. Not all fats are created equal, though. Below is a list of the best fats and the ones to avoid.

Best Fats

- **Animal fats** such beef tallow, lard, chicken schmaltz, duck fat: rich in vitamins and MCT oil.

- **Avocado oil:** rich in oleic acid, which is an omega-9 fatty acid. High in lutein, which is important for eye health.

- **Avocados:** rich in monounsaturated fats, which raise the level of good cholesterol while lowering the bad. They are also high in vitamin E, potassium, and fiber.

- **Coconut manna:** high in calcium, magnesium, and amino acids.

- **Coconut oil:** rich in medium-chain triglycerides (MCTs), which are a short-chain saturated fat, making it very easy to digest.

- **Eggs (pasture-raised):** contains choline, which is great for the brain, vitamins D and E, and high levels of omega-3 fatty acids.

- **Extra-virgin olive oil:** high in antioxidants and great for heart health.

- **Fatty fish such as salmon and sardines:** rich in heart-healthy omega-3 fatty acids.

- **Ghee:** clarified butter that has the milk solids removed. High in vitamins A and E.

- **Nuts and seeds:** rich in omega-3 fats, which help lower bad cholesterol.

Fats to Avoid

- **Corn oil, canola oil, soybean oil, and peanut oil:** highly refined, high in omega-6 fats, which can be inflammatory, and lacking in omega-3s. These are also from genetically modified (GMO) crops.

- **Margarine and shortening:** high in trans fats, which can increase the risk of heart disease.

SWEETENERS

For paleo sweetness, stick to natural options and avoid sweeteners that are artificial or highly processed.

Sweeteners to Have

- **Coconut sugar:** contains iron, zinc, calcium, and potassium and has a lower glycemic index than table sugar.
- **Dates:** good source of iron, potassium, and fiber.
- **Date sugar:** the granulated version of dates.
- **Dried fruit** with no added sugar: high in fiber and antioxidants, especially polyphenols, which can improve blood flow and help with better digestive health.
- **Honey:** rich in antioxidants and has antibacterial properties. It is important to note that honey should not be given to infants under one year old.

- **Maple sugar:** the granulated version of maple syrup.
- **Molasses:** contains iron, calcium, magnesium, selenium, and vitamin B_6.
- **Pure maple syrup:** great source of manganese, zinc, calcium, magnesium, and potassium.

Sweeteners to Avoid

- **Agave:** This is usually marketed as "natural," but it is highly processed and composed mainly of fructose (even more than high-fructose corn syrup), which is associated with fatty liver disease and type 2 diabetes.
- **Artificial sweeteners (aspartame, sorbitol, mannitol, Splenda, xylitol, Sweet'N Low, sucralose, Equal):** can cause gas, bloating, cramping, diarrhea, and acid reflux. Also linked to high blood pressure, heart disease, and diabetes.

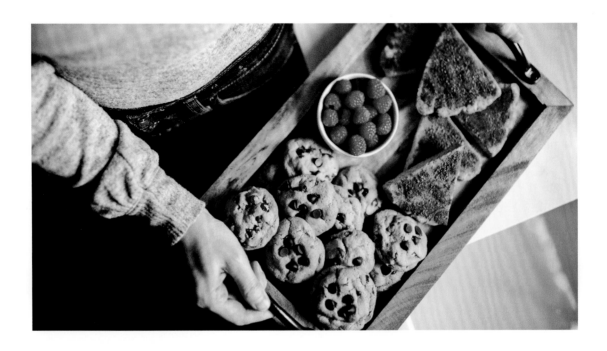

- **Erythritol:** Some people consider this paleo because it's not artificial, but it's a sweetener that is derived from cornstarch, which is not paleo. It can also cause digestive issues such as gas and bloating.

- **High-fructose corn syrup:** an artificial sweetener made from corn syrup shown to drive inflammation, which is associated with an increased risk of cancer, diabetes, obesity, and heart disease.

- **White/granulated sugar:** refined of all the natural components except the sucrose, and feeds the bad bacteria in your gut.

What Foods Should I Avoid?

Paleo is meant to be a gut-healing diet. By removing the foods that are hard on the gut, you are giving yourself a chance to heal and feel better.

Try not to focus on what you can't have, but rather what you can have. Switching from a Standard American Diet (SAD) to paleo may seem like a big adjustment because the SAD is centered around the foods in the list below. It may take a little while to relearn how to cook and shop, but in time it will become second nature.

- **Artificial sugar:** This includes sweeteners such as aspartame, xylitol, sucralose, and saccharin.

- **Dairy:** Lactose is not well tolerated by most people, and the protein in it is known to cause acne for those who are sensitive. Grass-fed butter is sometimes accepted in the paleo lifestyle, but do what works for you. I suggest ghee over butter because the milk solids (lactose) and casein have been removed.

Most people who are sensitive to dairy can handle ghee. Some good dairy-free alternatives are coconut milk and yogurt, almond milk, and homemade nut cheese.

- **Gluten:** Gluten is hard to digest and can cause gut inflammation in up to 80 percent of people. Common issues with gluten are GI disorders, mental health issues, skin conditions, and autoimmune disease. It can hide in sauces, dressings, processed meats, soups, and broths. Be sure to read labels carefully or buy products that you know are gluten free.

- **Grains:** This includes gluten-free grains such as oatmeal, quinoa, rice, millet, and buckwheat.

- **Legumes (including peanuts):** Legumes contain lectins, which can damage the lining of your intestines, causing inflammation. When your intestines are inflamed, their ability to absorb nutrients decreases.

- **Processed food:** Anything with a long list of ingredients that contain gluten, dairy, soy, or sugar. Common examples are packaged cookies, crackers, and yogurts. There are a lot of great paleo products that have come out recently, including granola, bars, dressings, and even frozen meals, but for the most part, focusing on veggies, fruit, and meats is the best.

- **Soy:** Soy is genetically modified and contains high levels of pesticides. It has a high concentration of goitrogens, which block the production of thyroid hormones. Most importantly, it contains estrogen-like chemicals that can raise estrogen levels and lower testosterone levels. For men, that means lower libido, fat accumulation around the waist, loss of energy and stamina, and man boobs. For women, it means disruption to the menstrual cycle and fertility and increased risk for breast cancer. For baby boys, it can mean too little testosterone, which can lead to failure to thrive, problems with puberty, lack of facial hair, and under-developed testicles.

- **Sugar:** Also known as dextrose, fructose, glucose, lactose, nectar, sucrose, malt, maltose, barley, and rice syrup.

- **Thickeners:** This includes carrageenan, guar gum, xanthan gum, gellan gum, dipotassium phosphate, and locust bean gum. These are all inflammatory, can cause gas and bloating, and are irritating to the gut. Paleo is meant to heal the gut, and these are doing the opposite. These thickeners are found in almond (and other nut) milks, canned coconut milk, dairy-free yogurt, ice cream, baked goods, grain-free bread and tortillas, sauces, dressings, and protein powders.

Saving Money

Paleo often gets a reputation as an expensive diet to follow, and it can be if you're buying all the fun packaged items, treats, and prepared food. It's great that those products are available, but if you're trying to save money, buy those items sparingly. Making your own mayonnaise, barbecue sauce, and banana bread is much more affordable than buying them.

One way to save money on produce is to buy what is in season. Not only will the food taste better, but it is also much more affordable.

Buy pantry items online. I often buy pantry staples such as canned tomatoes, nut butters, coconut flour, and nuts online because they are much cheaper than they are in stores.

Shop the local farmers' market if you have one available. This is a good way to get great deals on fresh produce and meat.

Stock up when there is a sale. If your local store has a great deal on a product you use often, buy extra and store it. This may mean freezing it if it's a fresh product. I find I do this most with pantry items, such as coco-nut oil, ghee, marinara sauce, tomatoes, and maple syrup. I do like to get meat that has been marked down and put it in the freezer right away. This will help me make quick meals later.

Plan ahead and make meals at home. This habit takes a little time to develop, but once you start making it a priority, it will save time and money. You can do what works best for you. Some people like meal prepping lots of food on a certain day and having it all week, and others just like to plan out the meals for the week. Either way, you are set up for success and won't feel tempted to hit a fast food restaurant on the way home from work. I like to write down the recipes I'm going to make, check which ingredients I already have, and then make a grocery list. I'm not one to make all the meals at once, but I love prepping ingredients ahead. Chopping veggies for a dish, cutting chicken into small pieces, and mixing spice mixes ahead of time all make the meal come together much quicker the day I make it. And that will save you money and stress.

Learning to Read Labels and Ingredient Lists

More paleo products are becoming available, and some foods that aren't labeled paleo are still compliant. Reading ingredient lists is an important part of living a paleo lifestyle. The front of packages can be misleading. The nutrition facts aren't super important, as counting calories, fat, and carbs aren't necessary, but you can check them for added sugar. The most important thing is to check ingredients to see whether there are any unwanted ones, such as sugar (in any form), canola oil, gums, or preservatives. (See pages 15–16 for more.) It will feel like a lot of reading at first, but you'll start to learn which products are compliant and which ones aren't, so it won't always be as time-consuming.

Sometimes you have to read the ingredient label to find the truth. Here are some examples I've found:

- Date sugar that had oat flour mixed in, but the front didn't state that. The oat flour makes it not paleo.

- A lot of almond and other nut butters have oils and sugar added to them.

- Vitamins can contain soy, wheat, and dairy. This surprised me when I first started reading the labels! Look for brands that specifically say they are free of soy, wheat, dairy, and gluten.

WHAT DO LABELS MEAN?

It can be confusing when you are first learning how to read labels. Companies put many labels on their packages; some are important and others not so much. Here is what to look for.

BEEF

- **100% grass fed:** Cows eat what their bodies are designed to eat, they are treated humanely, they graze freely outdoors, and they never eat grains.

- **Grass fed:** This one is trickier. It can mean they ate grass most of their lives and then finished with grain, or it might mean they ate a small amount of grass so it can technically be labeled that way.

- **Organic:** The animals must be fed a certain amount of organic food in their lives and have year-round outdoor access. All organic food is non-GMO, which is good, and it also means the cows didn't have any hormones, antibiotics, or drugs. The downside is the feed is still corn and grain. The organic label also doesn't mean the cow was treated humanely.

CHICKEN

- **Natural:** This label doesn't mean much, but it does mean that the chicken was minimally processed and doesn't contain artificial colors or flavors.

- **Non-organic:** The hens' feed contains soy, grain, and antibiotics. No outdoor space is provided for them. Hormones are not legal for any animal, so organic or not, no hormones are added.

- **Organic:** Must be naturally raised and free ranging. Their feed is non-GMO and no antibiotics are allowed, but it is still soy and corn. Organic is the most comprehensive label because it covers feed and living conditions. Look for certified organic.

- **Free range:** This label means the poultry had some outdoor access, but there is no set amount of time for free ranging. This also does not affect their feed, so they could be fed non-organic feed with antibiotics added.

- **Pasture raised:** The chickens are allowed to roam freely. They forage for food, but supplement with grain when food is less abundant. Because these birds move around naturally, their breasts are smaller and their legs are larger.

Labels That Are Misleading

- **Cage free:** All hens are cage free, so this doesn't mean anything.

- **No added hormones:** The FDA banned use of hormones in the 1950s.

- **100% vegetarian feed:** This just means the animals were fed no animal by-products. Is this important, though? No, chickens naturally eat bugs and worms if they are free to roam. This is a sure sign that these chickens were given no outdoor access.

PORK

- **Conventional:** Animals were fed grain, soy, and corn, which is not their natural diet, and the crops were sprayed with pesticides. They were given antibiotics and dewormers.

- **Organic:** Animals were given food that is organic, which means it's not genetically modified, but still corn, grain, and soy. Use of antibiotics is not allowed. Their worms are treated with natural remedies when needed.

- **Pasture raised:** When pigs are raised on a pasture, they get lots of sunshine, they can forage for food, and they can move around as intended. Because they are not living too closely with one another, they usually don't need antibiotics.

Labels to Look For

- **Antibiotic Free:** If it's organic, then it is already, but if it's non-organic, this is a good label.

- **Certified Organic**

- **American Humane Certified**

- **Animal Welfare Approved**

- **Global Animal Partnership**

SEAFOOD

- **Farm raised:** Commercially raised in confined areas such as tanks. They are bred to make the fish cheaper and more readily available. They are fed a mix of corn, grains, and a fishmeal that includes food coloring to give their flesh more color. Can be given antibiotics.

- **Wild caught:** They have a more diverse diet, resulting in better taste. They contain no antibiotics, because they are not at risk for disease like the farm-raised animals that live in confined areas. They have a darker pink color from the food they eat.

EGGS

- **Conventional:** Hens are confined to 64-square-inch (163 cm^2) cages, they never see daylight, and their diet is corn and soy.

- **Cage free:** Hens do not live inside wired cages, but they never go outside. They have just 18 square inches (46 cm^2) per bird and are always inside the barn. There is little ability to engage in natural behavior. They consume a corn and soy diet.

- **Standard free range:** Certified Humane standards requires only 24 square inches (61 cm^2) per bird. They must have outdoor access, but this might just be a "pop hole" they can stick their head through. They are fed a diet containing soy and corn. If you do choose these, look for the Certified Humane label, which means they meet specific pasture standards.

- **Organic:** To be USDA-certified organic, farms must be herbicide and pesticide free for at least a three-year period, and the hens must be fed an organic diet. This does not have any effect on the hens' quality of life.

- **Pasture raised:** This requires 108 square feet (33 m^2) per hen, and hens must be outdoors year-round with housing available to protect themselves. They eat worms, grass, and bugs, just like they are meant to.

What Is Low FODMAP?

After a couple of years of eating paleo, my ex-husband was still not feeling total relief digestively. I know he has irritable bowel syndrome (IBS), so I looked into diets that help symptoms of IBS and came across low FODMAP. FODMAP is an acronym that stands for "fermentable, oligo-, di, mono-saccharides, and polyols." These are the short-chain carbohydrates rich in fructose that are inefficiently absorbed in the small intestine. Every food has a different level of FODMAP from none to low, moderate, and high. People with leaky gut, IBS, small intestinal bacterial overgrowth (SIBO), and fibromyalgia can benefit from this diet to help with their gastrointestinal symptoms.

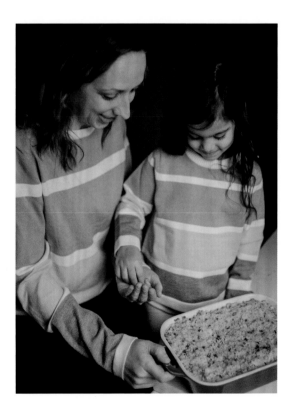

He got immediate relief as soon as I eliminated high-FODMAP foods. He has been eating this way for more than three years now, and he has reintroduced some foods, but still sticks to mostly low FODMAP. Along the way, I discovered I don't tolerate onion and garlic, so I avoid them and find other ways to get those flavors. I eat a lot of low FODMAP because that's the way I feel the best, but I can have some higher FODMAP foods and tolerate them.

I am including low-FODMAP recipes in this book because I know there are others who struggle with digestive issues even after starting to eat paleo. When looking for low-FODMAP recipes, I had trouble finding ones that were grain free, dairy free, and legume free. Most used non-paleo ingredients. I have learned to create flavorful, paleo, low-FODMAP recipes that many people enjoy. On those recipes, I include notes for making them not low FODMAP if you don't need to follow those guidelines. If you suspect you are sensitive to FODMAPs, try eliminating them for at least 30 days. You will feel immediate relief if you are sensitive.

Low FODMAP is not meant to be followed forever. It's an elimination diet to let your body heal. Then you can reintroduce some of the items slowly.

LOW-FODMAP FOODS (SAFE TO EAT)

- Alfalfa
- Avocado oil
- Bacon (sugar free)
- Bamboo shoots
- Banana, ripe
- Bean sprouts
- Bell peppers (not green)
- Blueberry
- Bok choy
- Cantaloupe
- Carrot
- Cassava/yuca
- Cherry tomatoes
- Chives
- Coconut oil
- Cucumber
- Dried herbs
- Eggplant
- Eggs
- Endive
- Fish and seafood
- Fresh herbs
- Garlic-infused oil
- Ghee
- Ginger
- Grapefruit
- Green beans
- Green onion, green part only
- Homemade mayonnaise
- Honeydew melon
- Kale
- Kiwi
- Lard
- Lemon
- Lettuce
- Lime
- Macadamia oil
- Mandarin orange
- Meat
- Olive oil
- Olives (check ingredients for onion and garlic)
- Orange
- Papaya
- Parsnip
- Passionfruit
- Pineapple
- Plantains
- Poultry
- Raspberry
- Rhubarb
- Rutabaga
- Salt and pepper
- Seaweed, nori
- Spices (not blends)
- Spinach
- Strawberry
- Swiss chard
- Tea (green, oolong, black, Yerba mate, rooibos)
- Tomatoes
- Turnip
- Vinegars
- White potatoes
- Zucchini

MODERATE-FODMAP FOODS (BE CAREFUL)

- Avocado
- Banana, unripe
- Beet
- Broccoli
- Brussels sprouts
- Butternut squash
- Cauliflower
- Celery
- Cocoa powder, unsweetened
- Coconut flour
- Coconut milk
- Coconut sugar
- Coffee
- Dried coconut
- Dry wines
- Fennel
- Grapes (10 per serving)
- Green peas
- Guacamole
- Lychee
- Macadamia nuts
- Maple syrup
- Mushrooms
- Pecans
- Pine nuts
- Pumpkin seeds
- Sauerkraut
- Sesame seeds
- Sunflower seeds
- Sweet potatoes
- Walnuts

HIGH-FODMAP FOODS (AVOID)

- Agave
- Almond
- Any processed meat containing onion and garlic, such as hot dogs, sausages, meat sticks, jerky
- Apple
- Apricot
- Artichoke
- Artificial sweeteners
- Asparagus
- Blackberries
- Cabbage
- Cashews
- Cherries
- Dried fruits
- Fruit juice
- Garlic
- Garlic powder
- Grapes (more than 15)
- Gums, carrageenan and other thickeners
- Hazelnuts
- Honey
- Leeks
- Mango
- Nectarine
- Okra
- Onion powder
- Onions
- Peach
- Pear
- Persimmon
- Pistachios
- Plum
- Port wines
- Radicchio
- Shallot
- Snow peas
- Sugar-free treats
- Sugar snap peas
- Sweet wines
- Tomato sauces and paste
- Watermelon

Chapter 2

must-have paleo kitchen tools

H ere are some of the basic tools you'll want to have on hand when planning and cooking the recipes in this book.

- **Baking pans:** You'll need a 9 by 9-inch (23 by 23 cm) for desserts or small casseroles and a 13 by 9-inch (33 by 23 cm) for bigger casseroles and cooking meat.

- **Cutting boards:** You'll need at least two, one for fruit and veggies and one for meat.

- **Deep-dish pie pan:** This is great for pie of course, but also egg bakes.

- **Frying pans:** Have at least two, a smaller one and a larger one. A 6- to 8-inch (15–20 cm) pan is great for making eggs, and a 10- to 12-inch (25–30 cm) pan is handy for browning meat or cooking veggies. Look for stainless steel or cast iron, and try to avoid nonstick pans, because they can contain toxic chemicals that should be avoided.

- **Glass measuring cup:** This is needed for properly measuring liquids.

- **Kitchen scale:** This is great for weighing ingredients when needed. A scale isn't as important for cooking as it is for baking, which needs to be more exact.

- **Knives:** You'll need a paring knife for cutting hard squash as well as smaller tasks such as prepping vegetables and slicing fruit. A large chef's knife is great for chopping nuts.

- **Ladle:** This is for serving soup.

- **Large stockpot:** This is my go-to for making soups.

- **Loaf pan:** This is for breads and desserts such as fudge.

- **Mason jars:** These are great for storing homemade sauces and dressings. Smaller ones can hold seasonings.

- **Measuring cups:** These are needed for measuring dry ingredients. Usually they come in ¼-, ⅓-, ½-, and 1-cup (60, 80, 120, and 240 ml) measurements.

- **Measuring spoons:** These come in sets of ¼ teaspoon, ½ teaspoon, 1 teaspoon, and 1 tablespoon (15 ml).

- **Meat thermometer:** This is so important for making sure chicken is cooked through and pork is done to your desired temperature.

- **Metal whisk:** This is great for making sure no lumps are in the mixture you are making.

- **Microplane or zester:** This is great for desserts, sauces, and dishes with citrus or ginger.

- **Mixing bowls:** Have at least two, so when making desserts you can have both going, but a couple more isn't a bad idea. I don't just use mine for desserts, though; I mix casserole ingredients and meatball mixtures in them, and I place cut veggies in them before use in a recipe.

- **Muffin tin:** This can be used for sweet or savory dishes.

- **Parchment paper:** Technically this isn't a tool, but it's something that is always great to use. It makes cleanup so easy and prevents food from sticking to the pan. This is especially important for egg dishes—they tend to stick the worst!

- **Rimmed baking sheets:** A few different sizes are nice to have for different needs. A half sheet is best for cookies, meatballs, and meatloaf. A quarter sheet is best for roasting a small amount of vegetables or rewarming food in the oven. Try to avoid nonstick for these.

- **Spatulas:** A must for baking to scrape the bowl clean.

- **Stainless steel saucepans:** The 1- and 2-quart (1 and 2 L) sizes are my most commonly used saucepans. These are great for making hot chocolate and sauces, melting chocolate, and making sweetened condensed milk.

- **Tongs:** I use these most for removing food from the pressure cooker and meat from soups to chop or shred.

- **Turner:** This is great for making pancakes, of course, but also serving casseroles.

- **Vegetables peeler:** I leave the skin on a lot of veggies such as potatoes and carrots, but a peeler comes in handy for butternut squash and cucumbers.

- **Wire cooling rack:** This is great to use on top of a baking sheet when baking coated food to get even cooking on all sides.

- **Wooden spoons:** These are my favorite tool for mixing desserts!

You can definitely eat paleo with these basics, but there are also some appliances that will make your life so much easier and more enjoyable. Here is what I have and love.

- **Electric hand mixer:** This is great for making desserts and whenever you need to mix the ingredients really well. It's less expensive and takes up less space than a stand mixer.

- **Enamel-coated cast-iron Dutch oven:** This is great for roasts, whole chickens, soups, and skillet meals. It is more expensive than a traditional stockpot, but it will last your whole life.

- **Glass storage containers:** Glass is great for storing leftovers because it doesn't hold color or flavor and cleans easily. Most glass storage containers can be frozen, microwaved, cleaned in the dishwasher, and used to bake in the oven. Having a set of multiple sizes is great for storing different items. You could use small ones for prepped veggies and larger ones for soups, for example.

- **High-powered blender or food processor:** This is great for making soups, your own nut milks, and desserts for which you are blending dates with nuts. These can vary in price from $150 to more than $700, so just get one that works in your budget.

- **Ice cream maker:** This is maybe not a must, but it's an affordable addition to your appliances that results in pure deliciousness. Homemade ice cream is super simple to make, and you can control the ingredients going in, meaning it can be dairy free and naturally sweetened.

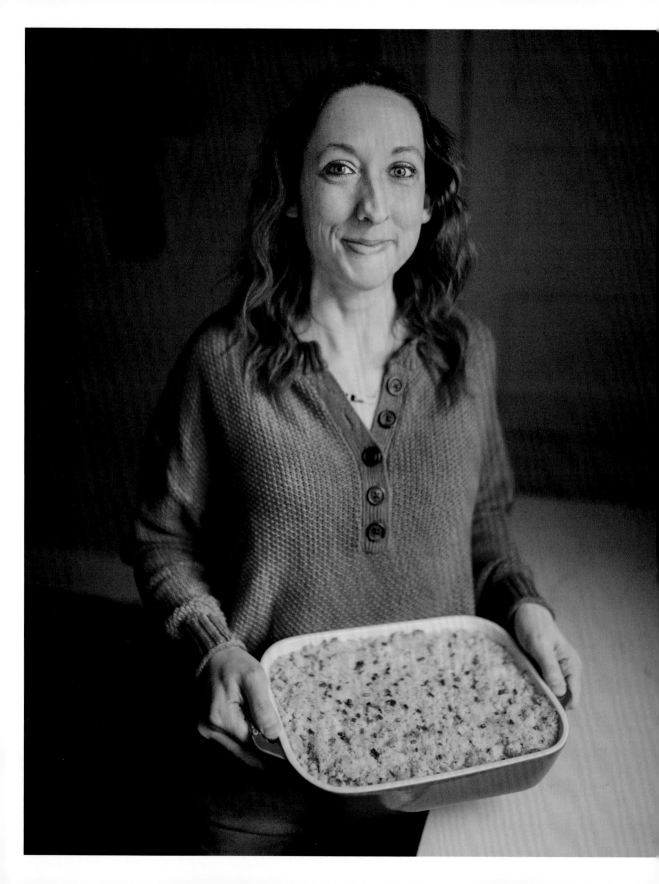

- **Immersion blender:** This is more affordable than a high-powdered blender and one of my most used tools. It can quickly make mayo, dressings, creamy soups, and fruit and almond milk smoothies.

- **Instant Pot or electric pressure cooker:** I didn't include many pressure cooker recipes because I know not everyone has one, but this is such a great tool for making quick meals. I got mine when my daughter was a baby, and it was a complete lifesaver for making sure meals were still being made.

- **Spiral vegetable slicer:** Finding veggie "noodles" premade in the store is common, but they are more affordable and last longer when you make them yourself. Zucchini is the most common "noodle," but you can also make them from cut sweet potato, carrot, apple, cucumber, white potato, and the neck of a butternut squash. Bell peppers and onions can be cut on this as well; they will just slice, not make noodles.

Stocking Your Kitchen for Success

Keeping a pantry and refrigerator stocked with paleo basics will help you whip up quick meals. You definitely want to focus on fresh ingredients, but having these essentials already on hand makes mealtime so easy.

FOR THE PANTRY: DRY GOODS

- **Almond flour:** Blanched is the best for baking and coating. This will not thicken sauces.
- **Arrowroot powder:** To thicken sauces.
- **Cacao powder**
- **Chocolate chips:** Unsweetened and coconut sugar sweetened (such as Santa Barbara).
- **Coconut flour:** For baking and coating meat; not good for thickening sauces.
- **Coconut sugar**
- **Coffee and tea**
- **Dates and dried fruit** (no sugar added)
- **Maple sugar**
- **Paleo pancake mix** (such as Birch Benders or Simple Mills)
- **Raw nuts and seeds**
- **Spices**

CANNED AND JARRED GOODS

- **BBQ sauce** (such as Primal Kitchen)
- **Diced green chiles**
- **Ghee**
- **Ketchup** (such as Primal Kitchen)
- **Mustard** (such as Annie's or Primal Kitchen)
- **Nut and seed butters** with one or two ingredients, just the nut and salt
- **Olives**
- **Paleo mayo** (such as Primal Kitchen)
- **Tomatoes,** diced fire-roasted
- **Tuna, salmon, and crab**

LIQUIDS

- **Bone broth:** This comes in handy for making soups and stews quickly. Look for versions made from grass-fed animals and check the ingredients for no added soy or sugar.

- **Coconut aminos:** This is the liquid made from the aged sap of coconut blossoms. It is a great soy sauce alternative, less salty and sweeter. Don't get this confused with liquid aminos, which are soy-based and not paleo. Coconut aminos can be found in most stores by the sauces or in the ethnic section.

- **Full-fat coconut milk:** Look for guar gum free. I love using this for homemade ice cream, in soups for creaminess, and to make sauces.

- **Honey:** Honey can be interchanged with maple syrup 1:1, but sometimes darkens in the baking process.

- **Maple syrup:** This is my most used sweetener for baked goods. It has a mild flavor and bakes well. This is 100% pure maple syrup, not pancake syrup, which is mostly high-fructose corn syrup.

- **Marinara sauce:** Such as Rao's Sensitive for low FODMAP or traditional marinara if you don't need low FODMAP. Check ingredient lists for no added canola oil or sugar.

- **Oils:** Avocado oil, extra virgin olive oil, toasted sesame oil, coconut oil, and garlic-infused olive oil. It's important to use a variety so you're getting fats from different sources.

- **Vinegars:** Coconut and apple cider. Use in sauces and dressings.

REFRIGERATOR

- **Almond milk:** Homemade or store-bought. Look for one with just two ingredients, almonds and water, so you know it's not mostly water and fillers. Avoid ones with carrageenan, gellan gum, locust bean gum, acacia gum, and dipotassium phosphate. (See page 16.)

- **Eggs:** Preferably pastured raised.

- **Fresh herbs:** Chives, rosemary, and thyme are my most used ones. They will elevate any meal.

- **Grass-fed hot dogs:** I like Teton Waters Ranch.

FREEZER

- **Chicken:** Breast, thighs, or whole.

- **Fruit:** Berries, apples, and pineapple.

- **Ground beef:** The start to the quickest meals.

- **Ground chicken and pork:** For homemade sausage and mixing with beef for meatballs.

- **Vegetables:** Green beans, broccoli, shredded potatoes, onions, and any other favorites. Riced cauliflower is very popular if you like making cauliflower rice.

Frequently Asked Questions on Paleo Baking

Paleo baking is much different than traditional baking. It's not hard once you learn about the different types of flours and how they work. Here are common questions I get.

CAN I SUBSTITUTE FOR ANOTHER FLOUR?

Most likely, no. You definitely cannot substitute coconut flour for any other flour. Coconut flour is unique in the fact that it's a dry flour and absorbs a lot of liquid. A small amount is needed in recipes. If it is substituted for almond flour, the result will be dry and crumbly. The recipes I create have been tested multiple times to get the exact measurements right; if they are changed, the dish may not turn out.

Cashew flour can be used in place of almond flour if you have an almond sensitivity.

Cassava flour is a popular nut-free flour, but it has a strong flavor and dense texture. Subbing it 1:1 is risky, and results are not guaranteed.

CAN I USE ANOTHER OIL?

Yes! I use ghee a lot for the buttery taste, but if you don't tolerate ghee, use refined coconut oil. I also like butter-flavored coconut oil because it still gives a buttery taste, but it's completely dairy free. I don't recommend vegan butter replacements because they are mostly water and can affect the outcome of the recipe.

CAN I USE A DIFFERENT SWEETENER?

Most likely, yes. You do need to stick to a similar sweetener—liquid for liquid and granulated for granulated. If you use honey in a recipe that calls for coconut sugar, for example, the end result will be too wet. Coconut sugar and maple sugar are interchangeable, and honey and maple syrup are interchangeable.

CAN I USE AN EGG REPLACEMENT?

Usually, yes. Especially for brownies, egg replacements work great. They may affect the rise of a cake or spreading of a cookie, but the taste should still be okay. I'm hesitant to recommend substituting for eggs in any recipe with three or more eggs, but it's your choice if you're willing to chance it. I know having an egg allergy can be hard to work around.

Egg replacements:

- **Chia egg:** 1 tablespoon (8 g) chia seeds mixed with 2½ tablespoons (37 ml) water. Let sit for 5 minutes to thicken.

- **Flax egg:** 1 tablespoon (12 g) flax seeds mixed with 2½ tablespoons (37 ml) water. Let sit for 5 minutes to thicken.

- **Gelatin egg:** 1 tablespoon (12 g) grass-fed beef gelatin mixed with 3 tablespoons (45 ml) warm to hot water. Stir until mixed well. Mixture will thicken. This is not a vegan option, but this replacement works great.

- **Mashed banana:** ¼ cup (58 g) mashed banana per egg. This will, of course, change the flavor of the recipe.

- **Unsweetened applesauce:** ¼ cup (60 g) applesauce per egg. This is a milder flavor than banana.

Recipes

Chapter 3

———

basics

These recipes are the basics that help meals come together quickly. Easily made with pantry staples, they may be recipes you have never thought to make yourself—like ketchup. But taking the time to do so is worth it. Homemade is always the freshest and most flavorful!

mayo

YIELD 1½ CUPS (354 ML)

PREP TIME 5 MINUTES

COOK TIME N/A

low LOW FODMAP, NUT FREE

1 large egg, at room temperature

1 tablespoon (15 ml) coconut vinegar or white vinegar

1 tablespoon (15 ml) lemon juice, ideally freshly squeezed

½ teaspoon salt

¼ teaspoon ground black pepper

1 cup (240 ml) avocado oil

Making your own mayo is quick and easy. This version is thick, creamy, mild in flavor, and made in just a couple of minutes. It uses ingredients you most likely have on hand, which means you can make it whenever it's needed. It's also more affordable than store-bought mayonnaise. I love using this for chicken salad and egg salad. It's also a great base for dips and dressings.

1. Place the egg, vinegar, lemon juice, salt, and pepper in a blender or a wide-mouth mason jar.

2. Process the ingredients in the blender, or with an immersion blender in the jar, until combined. With the blender on or the immersion blender running, slowly drizzle in the oil until the mixture is thick and creamy.

3. Move the immersion blender up and down in the jar until the mixture is thick. This should take less than a minute.

4. Store in the refrigerator for up to 2 weeks.

ketchup

YIELD 3 CUPS (710 ML)

PREP TIME 5 MINUTES

COOK TIME 30 MINUTES

EGG FREE, NUT FREE

½ cup (74 g) chopped pitted dates

One 6-ounce (170 g) can tomato paste, organic if possible

One 14.5-ounce (411 g) can diced tomatoes

2 tablespoons (30 ml) coconut vinegar or apple cider vinegar

½ cup (120 ml) bone broth or water

1 teaspoon garlic powder

1 teaspoon onion powder

1 teaspoon salt

¼ teaspoon cayenne pepper (optional)

You are going to be amazed at how good homemade ketchup can taste. It has a rich flavor and a little sweetness from the dates, and it tastes much fresher than the store-bought kind. Making it yourself means you have control over what goes in it—in fact, I like to use fire-roasted diced tomatoes for added flavor! It's also packed with all nourishing ingredients. This has converted many ketchup-haters into ketchup-lovers!

1. Place all the ingredients in a 2-quart (2 L) saucepan.

2. Cook, uncovered, over medium-low heat for 20 minutes. Turn off the heat. Puree the mixture with an immersion blender until smooth.

3. Continue to cook the ketchup, uncovered, over low heat for 10 minutes, until thick and smooth.

4. Let cool. Ladle into tightly covered jars and store in the refrigerator for 2–3 weeks.

low-FODMAP ketchup

YIELD 3 CUPS (710 ML)

PREP TIME 5 MINUTES

COOK TIME 20 MINUTES

EGG FREE, **low** LOW FODMAP, NUT FREE

Two 14.5-ounce (411 g) cans
fire-roasted diced tomatoes

¼ cup (60 ml) balsamic vinegar

¼ cup (60 ml) coconut aminos

2 tablespoons (30 ml) garlic-infused
olive oil

¾ teaspoon salt

¼ teaspoon ground black pepper

I came up with this recipe when my other ketchup recipe no longer worked for us, due to the dates, onion, and garlic. The balsamic vinegar gives this a great depth of flavor, and it comes together quickly.

1. Place all the ingredients in a medium-size saucepan. Blend with an immersion blender until smooth.

2. Cook, uncovered, over medium heat, stirring regularly, for 15–20 minutes, or until the ketchup thickens. Turn off the heat and blend again.

3. Let cool. Ladle into tightly covered jars and store in the refrigerator for 2–3 weeks.

barbecue sauce

YIELD 3 CUPS (710 ML)

PREP TIME 5 MINUTES

COOK TIME 20 MINUTES

EGG FREE, NUT FREE

One 6-ounce (170 g) can tomato paste

One 14.5-ounce (406 g) can fire-roasted diced tomatoes

½ cup (120 ml) coconut vinegar or apple cider vinegar

½ cup (78 g) pitted dates (about 8 Medjool dates)

½ cup (120 ml) bone broth or water

1 teaspoon garlic powder

1 teaspoon onion powder

1 teaspoon salt

½ teaspoon red pepper flakes

1 tablespoon chili powder

1 teaspoon yellow mustard

2 teaspoons smoked paprika

½ teaspoon hot sauce (optional)

3 tablespoons (39 g) coconut oil or (45 g) ghee

This barbecue sauce is so much better than the store-bought kind! It's thick, with a little spice, a little heat, and just a touch of smokiness. This is great brushed on chicken and ribs, paired with meatballs, or used as a dip for chicken. It can also be added to pulled pork or beef.

Note: Be sure to use a large saucepan—the sauce will splatter if you use a smaller one.

1. Place all the ingredients in a large saucepan and cook, uncovered, over medium heat for 10 minutes.

2. Turn off the heat and blend using an immersion blender. Alternatively, transfer to a blender and process on medium-high speed until smooth. If using a blender, remove the top piece on the lid and cover with a kitchen towel while blending.

3. Continue cooking for another 10 minutes, or until the sauce reaches your desired thickness. If it's too thick, add a little broth or water. If it's too thin, keep cooking.

4. Let cool. Ladle into tightly covered jars and store in the refrigerator for 2–3 weeks.

ranch dressing

YIELD 2 CUPS (473 ML)

PREP TIME 5 MINUTES

COOK TIME N/A

NUT FREE

1 cup (240 ml) mayonnaise, homemade (page 32) or paleo store-bought

One 13.5-ounce (378 ml) can coconut cream

1 teaspoon garlic powder

1 teaspoon onion powder

2 tablespoons dried parsley

½ teaspoon salt

¼ teaspoon ground black pepper

This thick and creamy dressing whisks together quickly and is great for dipping veggies in or topping a salad.

1. In a medium-size bowl, whisk the mayo and coconut cream until fully combined.

2. Add the garlic powder, onion powder, parsley, salt, and pepper. Whisk to combine. It will be pretty thin, but it will set up in the refrigerator.

3. Transfer to a tightly sealed container and store in the refrigerator for up to 2 weeks.

spaghetti squash

YIELD 4-6 SERVINGS

PREP TIME 8 MINUTES FOR THE PRESSURE COOKER OR 10 MINUTES FOR THE OVEN

COOK TIME 8-35 MINUTES

EGG FREE, **low** LOW FODMAP, NUT FREE

1 large (4- to 6-pound [1.8–2.7 kg]) spaghetti squash

½ teaspoon salt

This is one of my favorite veggies to use in casseroles or as a bed for meatballs. You have two options for how to cook it, in the oven or in a pressure cooker. Either way, it will come out perfectly tender with long strands. The oven method is nice when you have a little more time or don't have a pressure cooker. Using a pressure cooker is great because it is so quick and requires no oven heating. It's perfect for the warm months when you don't want the house warmed up.

OVEN

1. Preheat the oven to 425°F (220°C or gas mark 7). Line a baking sheet with parchment paper.

2. Place the spaghetti squash on a cutting board. Cut it in half lengthwise with a sharp knife. Each half will have an end piece. This is what creates the long strands that resemble spaghetti noodles. Cutting it the other way results in short noodles.

3. Scoop out all the seeds with a spoon and discard. Sprinkle a little salt on each spaghetti squash half and place them cut side down on the prepared baking sheet.

4. Bake for 30–35 minutes, or until the skin can be easily pierced with a fork.

5. Flip each spaghetti squash half over to release steam. Let cool for about 10 minutes. Pull the strands away from the skin using a fork.

PRESSURE COOKER

1. Follow steps 2 and 3 above.

2. Place the squash in the pressure cooker on a steam rack.

3. Add ¼ cup (60 ml) water, put the lid on, and make sure the valve is closed. Hit the manual button and set the time to 8 minutes.

4. Once done, hit Cancel to release the pressure and remove the squash with tongs.

5. Pull the strands away from the skin using a fork.

Recipes

Chapter 4

---

breakfast

The Standard American Diet breakfast consists of cereal, donuts, and toaster pastries. But rethinking and putting a little extra time into breakfast will make it satisfying and nourishing. Breakfast food that will truly fuel you will give you a great start to the day, and you will feel your best. I have sweet and savory options in this chapter, and most can be made ahead for busy mornings.

sausage gravy casserole

YIELD 4-6 SERVINGS

PREP TIME 20 MINUTES

COOK TIME 40 MINUTES

EGG FREE, **low** LOW FODMAP IF HOMEMADE SAUSAGE IS USED, NUT FREE IF COCONUT MILK IS SUBSTITUTED FOR ALMOND MILK

(IF YOU DON'T NEED LOW FODMAP, YOU MAY USE ALL GHEE INSTEAD OF A MIXTURE OF GARLIC-INFUSED OLIVE OIL AND GHEE AND A FEW CLOVES OF FRESH GARLIC, MINCED.)

One 1-pound (454 g) bag frozen hash browns

1 pound (454 g) breakfast sausage, homemade (page 54) or sugar-free store-bought

GRAVY

1 tablespoon (15 ml) garlic-infused olive oil

2 tablespoons (30 g) ghee

3 tablespoons (24 g) cassava flour

2½ cups (600 ml) almond milk

1 teaspoon dried sage

1 teaspoon fennel seeds

½ teaspoon salt

¼ teaspoon pepper

You are going to love this breakfast! It features a creamy gravy, homemade breakfast sausage, and shredded potatoes all baked into a delightful casserole.

1. Preheat the oven to 350°F (180°C or gas mark 4). Line a 9 by 9-inch (23 by 23 cm) baking pan with parchment paper. Place the frozen hash browns in a large bowl.

2. Cook the breakfast sausage in a large skillet over medium heat, breaking it into small pieces as it cooks, for 5–7 minutes. Add the sausage to the hash browns.

3. Make the gravy: Heat the oil and ghee in a large skillet over medium heat. Sprinkle in the cassava flour and whisk until combined. Once a paste forms, add the almond milk and whisk to combine. The mixture will turn smooth and start to thicken. Add the sage, fennel, salt, and pepper and continue to whisk. It should take 5–7 minutes to thicken.

4. Add the sauce to the hash browns and sausage and stir. Pour the mixture into the prepared pan and bake for 40 minutes. Serve warm.

5. Store leftovers, covered, in the refrigerator for up to 6 days.

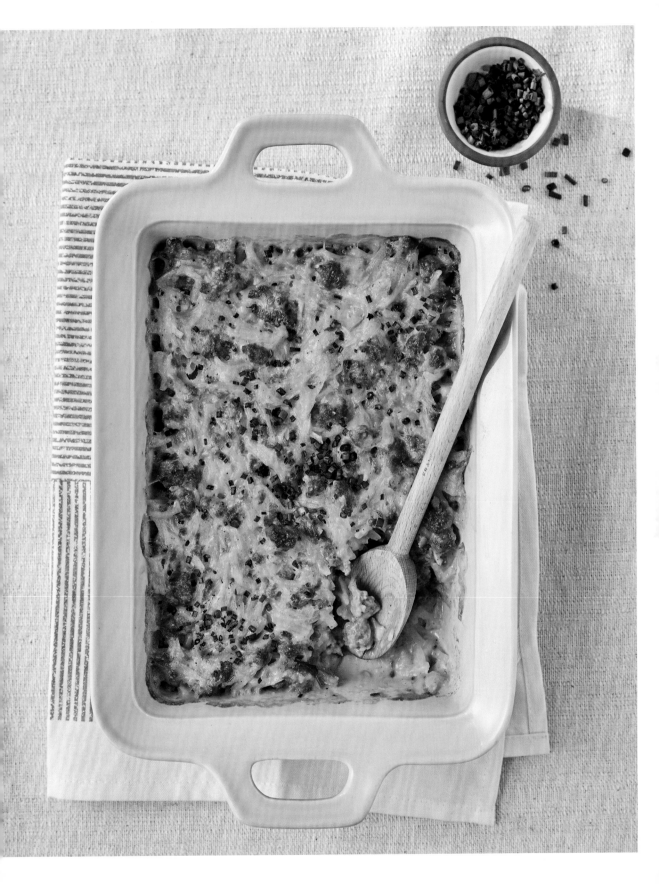

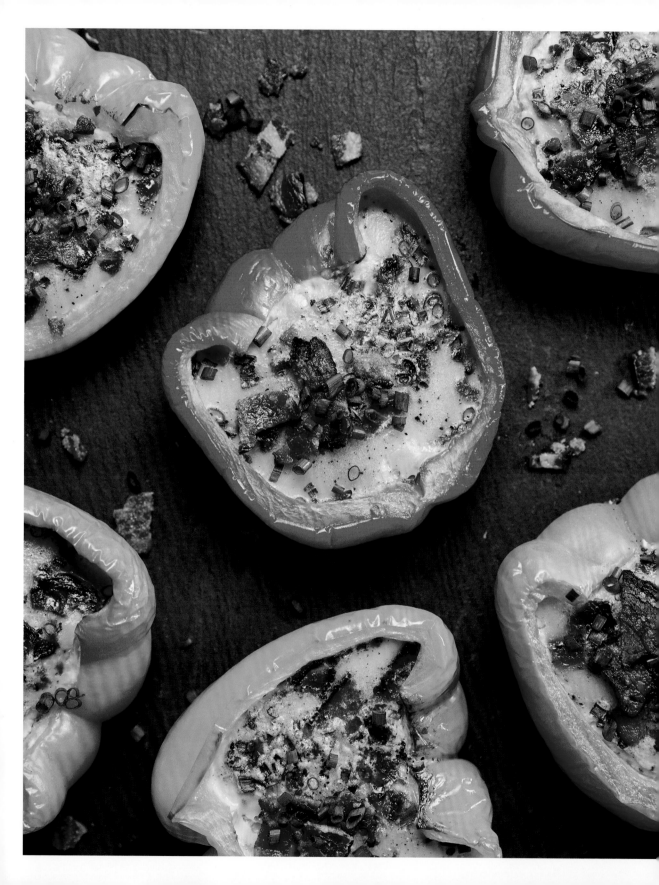

bell pepper egg boats

YIELD 5 SERVINGS

PREP TIME 10 MINUTES

COOK TIME 50 MINUTES

low LOW FODMAP IF GREEN BELL PEPPER ISN'T USED, NUT FREE IF COCONUT MILK IS USED

5 bell peppers, cut in half from top to bottom

1 tablespoon (15 ml) avocado oil

1 teaspoon salt, divided

10 large eggs

¼ cup (60 ml) almond milk

½ teaspoon ground black pepper

2 tablespoons (6 g) chopped chives

5 pieces bacon, cooked and crumbled, or substitute ½ pound (227 g) cooked breakfast sausage, homemade (page 54) or sugar-free store-bought

These boats are a fun breakfast that can be made ahead and enjoyed all week. They are super customizable—try adding in your favorite meat or veggies.

1. Preheat the oven to 375°F (190°C or gas mark 5).

2. Remove the stem and seeds from the peppers and place them in a 13 by 9-inch (33 by 23 cm) pan. Brush with the oil and sprinkle with ½ teaspoon (3 g) of the salt. Bake for 10 minutes.

3. While the peppers are baking, prepare the filling. Combine the eggs, remaining ½ teaspoon (3 g) salt, almond milk, pepper, chives, and bacon in a medium-size bowl. Mix until well combined.

4. Spoon mixture into the peppers' cavities, dividing as evenly as possible.

5. Bake for 35–40 minutes, or until the eggs have set. Serve warm.

6. Store leftovers, covered, in the refrigerator for up to 6 days.

kale and sausage egg bake

YIELD 6-8 SERVINGS

PREP TIME 25 MINUTES

COOK TIME 50 MINUTES

NUT FREE, **low** LOW FODMAP IF HOMEMADE SAUSAGE IS USED

1 pound (454 g) sweet potatoes, chopped into ½-inch (1 cm) chunks

2 tablespoons (30 ml) avocado oil, divided

½ teaspoon salt, divided

1 pound (454 g) breakfast sausage, homemade (page 54) or sugar-free store-bought

5 ounces (142 g) baby kale

12 large eggs

You can never have too many breakfast bake ideas! The sweet potato, sausage, and kale bake is hearty and nourishing.

1. Preheat the oven to 425°F (220°C or gas mark 7). Line a baking sheet with parchment paper. Line a 13 by 9-inch (33 by 23 cm) pan with parchment paper.

2. Place the sweet potatoes on the prepared baking sheet and toss with 1 tablespoon (15 ml) of the oil and ¼ teaspoon of the salt. Roast for 20 minutes, or until the potatoes are tender.

3. While the potatoes are cooking, cook the sausage in a large skillet over medium heat for 5–7 minutes, or until cooked through. Place the sausage in the prepared pan, spreading evenly.

4. Add the remaining 1 tablespoon (15 ml) oil to the skillet used for the sausage and add the kale. Sprinkle with the remaining ¼ teaspoon salt and cook for 2–3 minutes, or until tender. Spread the kale evenly over the sausage.

5. When the sweet potatoes are done roasting, place them in the pan with the kale and sausage and stir to combine. Reduce the oven temperature to 350°F (180°C or gas mark 4).

6. Crack the eggs into a medium-size bowl and whisk until well combined. Pour the eggs over the meat mixture. Stir a little if necessary, distributing the ingredients as evenly as possible.

7. Bake for 45–50 minutes, or until the middle is set. Serve warm.

8. Store leftovers, covered, in the refrigerator for up to 6 days.

breakfast burritos

YIELD 8 BURRITOS

PREP TIME 15 MINUTES

COOK TIME 20 MINUTES

8 grain-free tortillas*, such as Siete Almond Flour Tortillas

8 pieces sugar-free bacon

½ cup (75 g) diced red bell pepper, about half a large pepper

½ cup (80 g) diced onion, about half a medium onion

¼ teaspoon salt

2 tablespoons (30 ml) ghee

8 large eggs

¼ cup (60 ml) almond milk*

¼ teaspoon salt

¼ teaspoon black pepper

*THESE COULD BE NUT-FREE IF YOU FIND NUT-FREE TORTILLAS AND USE COCONUT MILK IN PLACE OF THE ALMOND MILK.

The dad of one of my high school friends made the best breakfast burritos and I always looked forward to them. Packed with all the fillings and so satisfying, these are a grain-free version, made with almond flour tortillas, but still just as delicious and comforting. They are pretty forgiving if you want to switch up the ingredients, just keep the measurements the same—and play around with your favorite fillings.

1. Cut bacon and cook in a large skillet over medium heat, stirring regularly, until crispy. About 10 minutes. Turn the heat off and remove from the pan and place on a plate.

2. Leave the bacon fat in the pan and add in the red pepper and onion. Turn heat back to medium and cook 5 minutes, until softened. Turn off the heat and remove the mixture to a bowl. Wipe down the pan and add the ghee.

3. In a large bowl, whisk together the eggs and almond milk. Turn the heat to medium and let the ghee melt. Add in the eggs and stir with a rubber spatula until fully cooked through, about 4 minutes. Add in the salt and pepper and mix well. Remove to a small bowl.

4. Assemble the burritos. Warm the tortillas so they are easy to fold. Baking them for 3 minutes in a 300°F (150°C or gas mark 2) oven works great.

5. Spread some eggs (about ¼ cup [55 g]) on the bottom, top with peppers and onion then top with the bacon. Fold to close. Repeat with the remaining.

6. Serve immediately or store in the fridge. Wrap in foil or wax paper to hold together.

chocolate chip muffins

YIELD 10 MUFFINS

PREP TIME 10 MINUTES

COOK TIME 27 MINUTES

These muffins are soft, moist, and loaded with chocolate chips. They are super easy to make with just a handful of ingredients, and they're a treat the whole family will love.

2 cups (224 g) almond flour

¼ cup (30 g) coconut flour

½ teaspoon baking soda

¼ teaspoon salt

⅓ cup (80 ml) maple syrup or honey

¼ cup (60 ml) melted ghee

3 large eggs, at room temperature

½ cup (85 g) dairy-free chocolate chips

1. Preheat the oven to 350°F (180°C or gas mark 4). Line a muffin pan with 10 parchment liners.

2. Combine the almond flour, coconut flour, baking soda, and salt in a large bowl. Stir well.

3. Add the maple syrup, ghee, and eggs. Mix with a spoon until well incorporated with no remaining dry spots. Add the chocolate chips and stir again.

4. Divide the batter evenly among the 10 liners. Bake for 25–27 minutes, or until a toothpick inserted into the center of a muffin comes out clean. Serve warm or at room temperature.

5. Store leftovers, covered, at room temperature for 2 days, or longer in the refrigerator.

chocolate cereal

YIELD 6–8 SERVINGS

PREP TIME 10 MINUTES

COOK TIME 30 MINUTES

EGG FREE

1½ cups (224 g) raw sunflower seeds

1 cup (116 g) raw almonds

1 cup (112 g) raw pecans

½ teaspoon salt

½ cup (40 g) cacao powder

¼ cup (48 g) coconut sugar

6 tablespoons (89 ml) melted coconut oil

2 tablespoons (30 ml) maple syrup

This cereal is very reminiscent of a popular chocolate cereal. It's crunchy and sweet, and makes a great snack.

1. Preheat the oven to 300°F (150°C or gas mark 2). Line a baking sheet with parchment paper.

2. Place the sunflower seeds, almonds, and pecans in a food processor and chop finely.

3. Pour the mixture into a large bowl and add the salt, cacao powder, coconut sugar, coconut oil, and maple syrup. Mix well and scoop onto the baking sheet. Spread evenly.

4. Bake for 20 minutes. Stir and bake for 10 more minutes. Let cool. This is great with some almond milk poured over it. It's also good as a snack by itself.

5. Store leftovers, covered, at room temperature for up to 10 days.

maple pecan "oatmeal"

YIELD 4–6 SERVINGS

PREP TIME 5 MINUTES

COOK TIME 40 MINUTES

low LOW FODMAP IF DIVIDED INTO 6 SERVINGS

2 tablespoons (15 g) coconut flour

1 cup (80 g) unsweetened shredded coconut

1 cup (112 g) raw pecans

1 large egg

⅓ cup (80 ml) maple syrup

1 teaspoon ground cinnamon

½ teaspoon salt

¾ cup (180 ml) almond milk

2 tablespoons (30 ml) melted ghee

You will not miss oatmeal if you have this grain-free version! The coconut and pecans mimic the texture of oatmeal, and the flavor is incredible. This makes a great breakfast or dessert.

1. Preheat the oven to 325°F (170°C or gas mark 3). Line a 9 by 9-inch (23 by 23 cm) pan with parchment paper.

2. Combine the coconut flour, shredded coconut, and pecans in a food processor and process for less than 1 minute, or until the mixture is crumbly and all the pieces are similar in size.

3. Pour the mixture into a large bowl. Add the egg, maple syrup, cinnamon, salt, almond milk, and ghee. Mix well.

4. Scoop the mixture into the prepared pan and spread evenly. Bake for 35–40 minutes, or until the edges are lightly brown. Cut into slices and serve warm. Add a drizzle of maple syrup and a few fresh berries on top if desired.

5. Store leftovers, covered, in the refrigerator for up to a week.

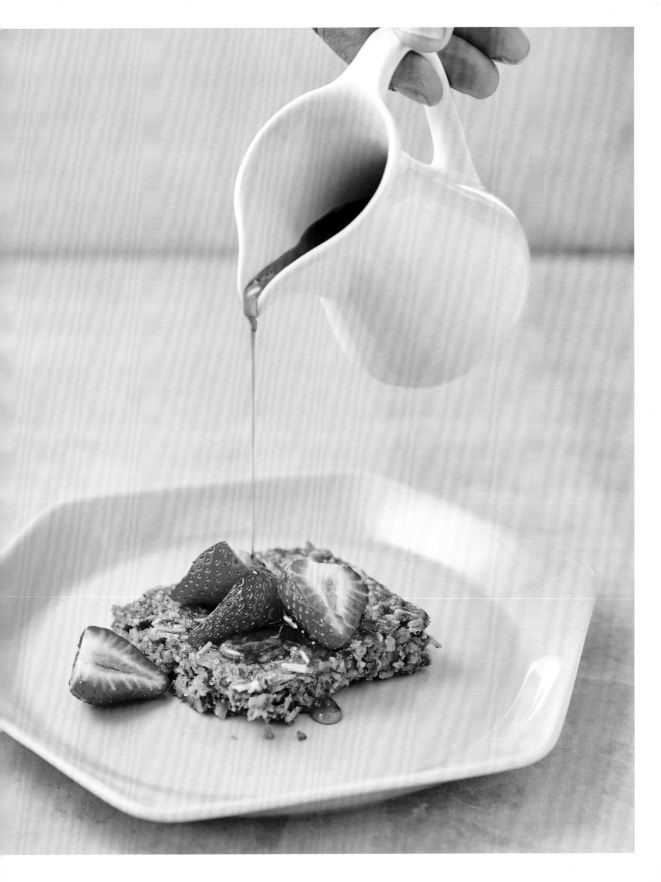

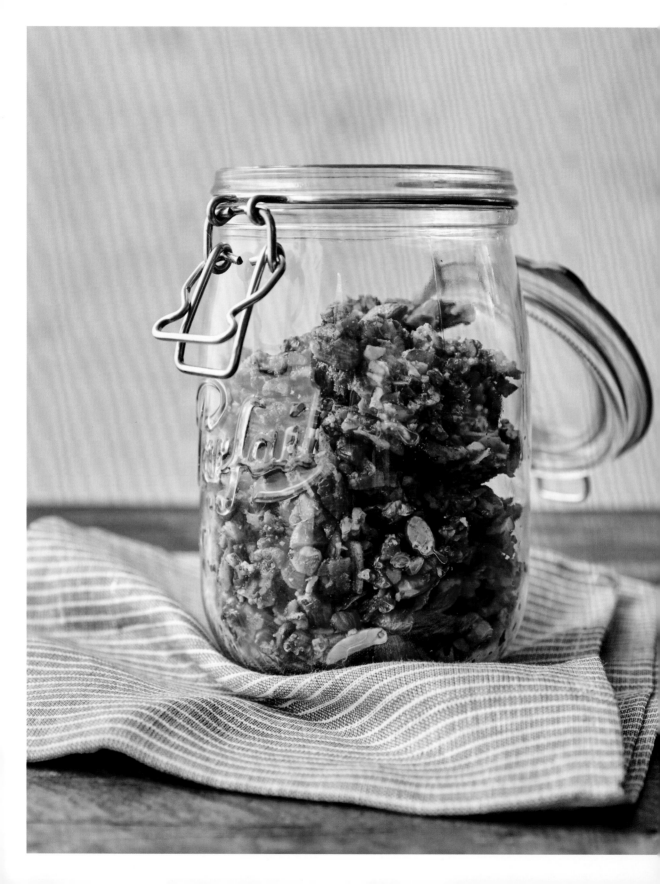

butter pecan granola

YIELD 6-8 SERVINGS

PREP TIME 10 MINUTES

COOK TIME 30 MINUTES

EGG FREE

1½ cups (168 g) raw pecan halves

1 cup (116 g) raw almonds

1 cup unsweetened (80 g) shredded coconut

½ teaspoon salt

1 teaspoon ground cinnamon

¼ cup (48 g) coconut sugar

½ cup (120 ml) melted ghee (or butter-flavored coconut oil)

2 tablespoons (30 ml) maple syrup

1 teaspoon vanilla extract

This granola has big clusters that are perfect for snacking or breakfast. It's crunchy, sweet, and so delish.

1. Preheat the oven to 300°F (150°C or gas mark 2). Line a baking sheet with parchment paper.

2. Blend the pecans, almonds, coconut, and salt in a food processor until the pieces are even in size. Transfer to a bowl. Add the cinnamon, coconut sugar, ghee, maple syrup, and vanilla. Stir well and spread evenly on the prepared baking sheet.

3. Bake for 25–30 minutes without stirring. Let cool without stirring and then break into clusters. This makes a great snack by itself or you can enjoy it with almond milk like cereal.

4. Store leftovers, covered, at room temperature for up to 10 days.

blueberry pancake bites

YIELD 24 MINI MUFFINS

PREP TIME 10 MINUTES

COOK TIME 18 MINUTES

NUT FREE

Tender pancakes topped with juicy blueberries make a perfect breakfast. And these have a fun mini size that is great for small hands!

4 large eggs, at room temperature

¼ cup (48 g) coconut sugar

½ cup (60 g) coconut flour

¼ teaspoon salt

1 teaspoon ground cinnamon

½ teaspoon baking soda

¼ cup (60 ml) melted ghee or butter-flavored coconut oil

2 tablespoons (60 ml) maple syrup

1 teaspoon vanilla extract

½ cup (74 g) blueberries

1. Preheat the oven to 325°F (170°C or gas mark 3). Line a mini muffin tin with 24 liners.

2. In a medium-size bowl, beat together the eggs and coconut sugar with a whisk. Add the coconut flour, salt, cinnamon, and baking soda and whisk again.

3. Add the ghee, maple syrup, and vanilla and stir with a wooden spoon. Scoop the mixture into the prepared muffin liners and top with 3 or 4 blueberries each. Bake for 18 minutes. Enjoy warm or at room temperature.

4. Store leftovers, covered, in the refrigerator for up to 5 days.

egg muffins

YIELD 12 MUFFINS

PREP TIME 20 MINUTES

COOK TIME 20 MINUTES

low LOW FODMAP, NUT FREE

These are handy for quick, on-the-go breakfasts. Make them ahead for easy mornings. Even with just a handful of ingredients, they are so delicious. The smoky bacon pairs wonderfully with the kale.

12 ounces (340 g) sugar-free bacon, cut into small pieces

5 ounces (142 g) baby kale or spinach

½ teaspoon salt

¼ teaspoon ground black pepper

12 large eggs

1. Preheat the oven to 375°F (190°C or gas mark 5). Line a muffin tin with 12 parchment liners.

2. Cook the bacon in a large skillet over medium heat for 10–12 minutes, or until crispy. Transfer to a large bowl, leaving the grease in the pan.

3. Add the kale to the bacon grease over medium heat, sprinkle with the salt and pepper, and cook for 3–4 minutes, or until wilted. Add the kale to the bowl with the bacon.

4. Break the eggs into the bacon mixture and stir well, making sure all the yolks are broken.

5. Scoop the mixture evenly into the parchment liners. Bake for 18–20 minutes, or until the eggs have set. Serve warm.

6. Store leftovers, covered, in the refrigerator for up to 6 days.

breakfast sausage

YIELD 9 PATTIES

PREP TIME 10 MINUTES

COOK TIME 10-15 MINUTES

low LOW FODMAP

No need to buy store-bought sausage when you can make it yourself! This sausage is tasty and simple. I love making a big batch and freezing it for later.

1 pound (454 g) ground turkey or pork

1 teaspoon salt

½ teaspoon ground black pepper

1 teaspoon (2 g) dried sage

½ teaspoon fennel seeds

¼ teaspoon red pepper flakes

2 teaspoons garlic-infused olive oil

2 teaspoons dried chives

1. Preheat the oven to 375°F (190°C or gas mark 5). Line a baking sheet with parchment paper.

2. Combine the ground turkey, salt, pepper, sage, fennel, red pepper flakes, garlic-infused olive oil, and chives in a large bowl. Mix well, making sure the seasonings are well distributed.

3. Scoop the mixture into ¼-cup (60 g) patties, making 9 total. Roll the patties into balls and press into ⅓ inch (8 mm)–thick circles.

4. Bake for 15 minutes. Alternatively, cook the turkey mixture in a medium-size skillet over medium heat, breaking it up as it cooks, for 7–10 minutes, or until fully cooked through.

5. Store leftovers, covered, in the refrigerator for up to a week. Breakfast sausage freezes well in a food-grade silicone bag. Let the sausage cool and then place it in the bag. Remove all the air from the bag and freeze for up to 6 months.

pumpkin pancake bake

YIELD 15 SERVINGS

PREP TIME 10 MINUTES

COOK TIME 33 MINUTES

1 cup (240 ml) canned pumpkin (not pumpkin pie filling)

4 large eggs, at room temperature

¼ cup (60 ml) melted ghee

½ cup (120 g) almond butter

¼ cup (60 ml) water

1 teaspoon vanilla extract

1¾ cups (196 g) almond flour

⅓ cup (40 g) coconut flour

½ cup (96 g) coconut sugar

1 teaspoon baking soda

2 teaspoons pumpkin pie spice

½ teaspoon ground cinnamon

¼ teaspoon salt

This is a quick way to make a big pancake. The recipe has no flipping, but the taste has all the yumminess of regular pancakes. Serve it with a drizzle of maple syrup.

1. Preheat the oven to 350°F (180°C or gas mark 4). Line a 13 by 9-inch (33 by 23 cm) pan with parchment paper or grease well with coconut oil.

2. Combine the pumpkin, eggs, ghee, almond butter, water, and vanilla in a large bowl. Stir well.

3. Combine the almond flour, coconut flour, coconut sugar, baking soda, pumpkin pie spice, cinnamon, and salt in a separate bowl. Stir to combine.

4. Add the dry ingredients to the wet ingredients and stir well, until no dry spots remain.

5. Pour the mixture into the prepared pan. Bake for 30–33 minutes, or until a toothpick inserted in the center comes out clean. Cut into squares and serve warm. This is great with a drizzle of maple syrup on top.

6. Store leftovers, covered, in the refrigerator for up to a week.

broccoli and ham crustless quiche

YIELD 4–6 SERVINGS

PREP TIME 25 MINUTES

COOK TIME 50 MINUTES

low LOW FODMAP, NUT FREE
IF COCONUT MILK IS SUBSTITUTED
FOR ALMOND MILK

12 ounces (340 g) frozen broccoli

1 tablespoon (15 ml) avocado oil

10 ounces (283 g) nitrate-free ham, chopped

¼ cup (24 g) chopped green onion

10 eggs

¼ cup (60 ml) almond milk

A few simple ingredients come together in this recipe to create a pleasing breakfast. This is great served with a side of fruit to make a complete meal.

1. Preheat the oven to 425°F (220°C or gas mark 7). Line a baking sheet with parchment paper. Grease a deep-dish pie plate well with coconut oil or line it with parchment paper.

2. Place the broccoli on the prepared baking sheet, drizzle with the avocado oil, and bake for 25 minutes, or until tender.

3. Place the ham and green onion in the prepared pie dish.

4. When the broccoli is done roasting, lower the oven temperature to 350°F (180°C or gas mark 4). Spread the broccoli evenly in the pie plate.

5. Combine the eggs and almond milk in a medium-size bowl. Stir until well mixed, with all the yolks broken. Pour the eggs over the ham mixture. Stir to make sure all the ingredients are distributed evenly.

6. Bake for 45–50 minutes, or until the center is set. Cut into slices and serve warm.

7. Store leftovers, covered, in the refrigerator for up to 6 days.

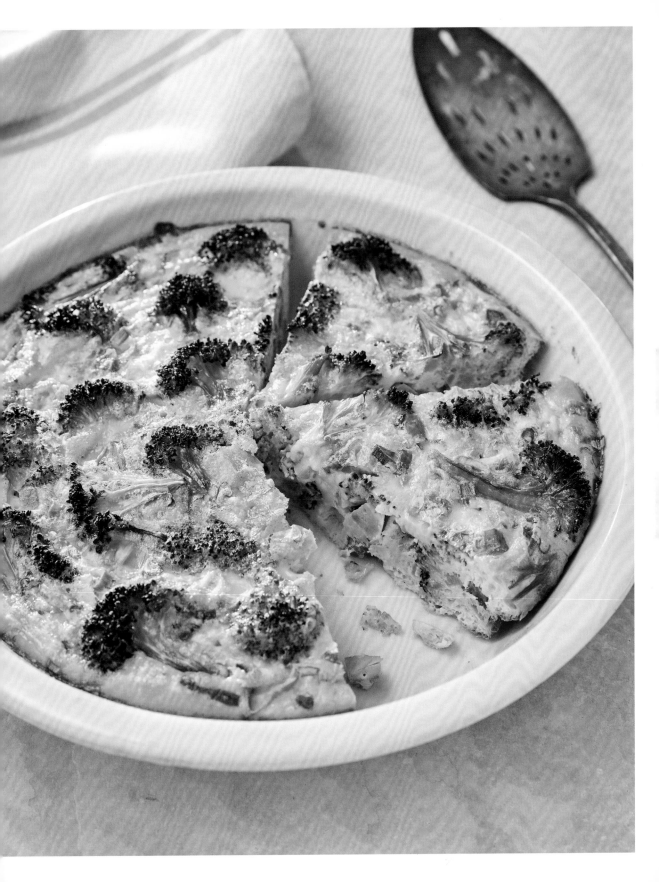

Recipes

Chapter 5

———

appetizers and sides

I am not big on throwing parties throughout the year, but I do love to offer appetizers at the holidays. These are some of my favorites to whip up—they are sure to be enjoyed. They are perfect for any party, gathering, or even family movie night. They're made with all real ingredients, but they're still fun and tasty.

hemp seed crackers

YIELD 50-60 CRACKERS

PREP TIME 10 MINUTES

COOK TIME 30 MINUTES

NUT FREE, <mark>low</mark> LOW FODMAP

(IF YOU DON'T NEED LOW FODMAP, YOU MAY USE 1 TEASPOON GARLIC POWDER IN PLACE OF THE OIL AND FEEL FREE TO ADD ½ TEASPOON ONION POWDER TO TASTE.)

1 cup (160 g) shelled hemp seeds

1 cup (149 g) raw sunflower seeds

1 large egg

1 tablespoon (15 ml) garlic-infused olive oil

2 teaspoons (5 g) Italian seasoning

¼ teaspoon salt

Making homemade crackers is easier than you think. These come out crunchy and are very hearty thanks to the seeds.

1. Preheat the oven to 300°F (150°C or gas mark 2). Line a baking sheet with parchment paper.

2. Combine the hemp seeds, sunflower seeds, egg, olive oil, Italian seasoning, and salt in a large bowl. Mix well.

3. Transfer the mixture to the prepared baking sheet and use your hands to press it into a 13 by 9-inch (33 by 23 cm) rectangle.

4. Bake for 20 minutes. Cut the crackers into 1-inch (3 cm) squares, separating them slightly, and bake for 10 more minutes.

5. Store leftovers, covered, at room temperature for up to 10 days.

zucchini tots

YIELD 15 SERVINGS

PREP TIME 15 MINUTES

COOK TIME 29 MINUTES

NUT FREE, **low** LOW FODMAP

(IF YOU DON'T NEED LOW FODMAP, YOU MAY USE ½ TEASPOON GARLIC POWDER IN PLACE OF THE GARLIC-INFUSED OLIVE OIL.)

2 cups (248 g) packed shredded zucchini (about 2 medium zucchini)

1 large egg

3 tablespoons (23 g) coconut flour

½ teaspoon salt

¼ teaspoon ground black pepper

1 teaspoon Italian seasoning

1 tablespoon (15 ml) garlic-infused olive oil

Here's a fun way to eat zucchini. These are handheld and lightly seasoned, and make a great snack or side dish.

1. Preheat the oven to 400°F (200°C or gas mark 6). Line a baking sheet with parchment paper.

2. Combine the zucchini, egg, coconut flour, salt, pepper, Italian seasoning, and oil in a large bowl. Mix with a wooden spoon until well combined.

3. Scoop into 1-tablespoon (15 g) balls and with your hands shape each into a tot shape, about 1½ inches (4 cm) long by 1 inch (3 cm) wide.

4. Bake for 12 minutes. Flip and bake for 12 more minutes. Bake for another 5 minutes if needed for tots to finish browning. Serve immediately. These are great dipped in paleo ranch dressing (page 36) or marinara sauce.

sweet potato fries with special sauce

YIELD 3-4 SERVINGS

PREP TIME 10 MINUTES

COOK TIME 30 MINUTES

EGG FREE IF THE SAUCE ISN'T USED, **low** LOW FODMAP, NUT FREE

(IF YOU DON'T NEED LOW FODMAP, YOU MAY ADD ¼ TEASPOON GARLIC POWDER TO THE SAUCE.)

1 large sweet potato

2 teaspoons (7 g) arrowroot powder/starch

1 tablespoon (15 ml) avocado oil

¼ teaspoon salt

SAUCE

⅓ cup (80 ml) mayonnaise, homemade (page 32) or paleo store-bought

¼ teaspoon chipotle powder

1 teaspoon garlic-infused olive oil

These sweet potato fries are crispy thanks to the arrowroot powder and salting after baking. The sauce has a little spice that tastes amazing with the potatoes' sweetness.

1. Preheat the oven to 425°F (220°C or gas mark 7). Line a baking sheet with parchment paper.

2. Cut the sweet potato into ¼-inch (6 mm) slices. (Note that I often like to cut the slices into ¼-inch [6 m] sticks.) Place them in a large bowl and toss with the arrowroot powder, trying to coat all the fries evenly. Leave any excess in the bowl. Arrange the fries in a single layer on the baking sheet. Drizzle with the avocado oil and toss to coat evenly. Do not salt at this point!

3. Bake for 15 minutes, remove from the oven and flip them, and then bake for another 15 minutes.

4. Remove from the oven and season with the salt.

5. Meanwhile, make the sauce: Place the mayo in a small bowl. Add the chipotle powder and olive oil. Stir well. Serve with the fries.

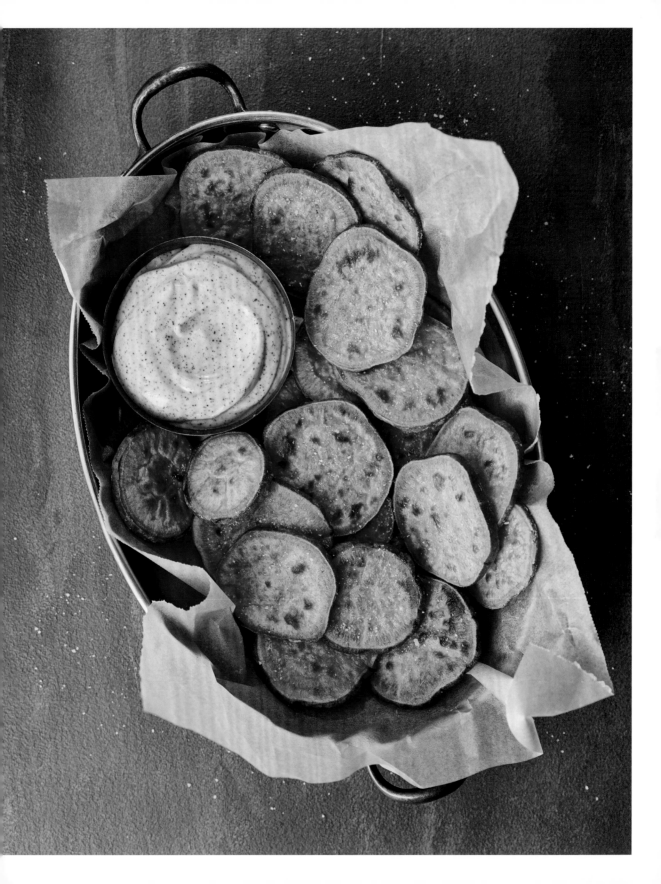

homemade applesauce

YIELD 8-10 SERVINGS

PREP TIME 20 MINUTES

COOK TIME 13 MINUTES FOR THE
PRESSURE COOKER OR 40 MINUTES
FOR THE STOVE

EGG FREE, NUT FREE

3 pounds (1.4 kg) apples

½ cup (120 ml) water

This recipe is simple, but special. My family made this applesauce a lot while I was growing up, and it always tastes better than store-bought. No added sugar is needed, and I encourage you to try a bowl warm—it's delightful. Add a little cinnamon if you like, and use whatever apples you love. The pressure cooker version creates a thinner applesauce, whereas the stovetop version is thick and chunky.

PRESSURE COOKER

1. Peel and core the apples and cut them into eighths. Place the apples pieces in the pressure cooker and add the water. Place the lid on and close the valve.

2. Cook on high for 8 minutes. Press Cancel and release the pressure. Press Sauté and cook for 3–5 minutes to thicken.

STOVE

1. Peel and core the apples and cut them into eighths. Place the cut apples in a large saucepan. Add the water, cover, and cook, stirring every 10 minutes, for 30 minutes. Mash with a spoon or a potato masher.

2. Cook for another 10 minutes if you prefer a thicker sauce. Turn off the heat. Let cool for chunky applesauce; blend for smooth applesauce. You can do this with an immersion blender right in the pan or pour the mixture into a blender and blend until smooth.

3. Serve warm or store leftovers, covered, in the refrigerator for up to a week.

garlic butter sautéed mushrooms

YIELD 4 SERVINGS

PREP TIME 10 MINUTES

COOK TIME 20 MINUTES

NUT FREE, EGG FREE

2 pounds (910 g) mushrooms, white or baby bellas

4 tablespoons (60 ml) ghee, divided

½ teaspoon salt

3 cloves minced garlic

1 tablespoon (2.4 g) fresh thyme

These mushrooms are quick to make and the perfect side to steak, chicken, or eggs. They are tender, flavorful, and the butter flavor comes from the ghee in this dish. The mushrooms can be prepped ahead and stored in the fridge if needed.

1. Wipe down the mushrooms with a damp cloth and cut into fourths.

2. Add 3 tablespoons (45 ml) of the ghee to a large skillet and turn heat to medium. Add in the mushrooms and cook for about 3 minutes, stirring to coat mushrooms in ghee. Let sit without stirring 7 minutes. During this time, the mushrooms will release a lot of moisture. Let that moisture cook off, stirring occasionally, which will take about 8 minutes.

3. Once the moisture has cooked off add the last tablespoon of ghee, garlic and thyme. Cook 2–3 minutes, until garlic is cooked and mushrooms are coated in the ghee.

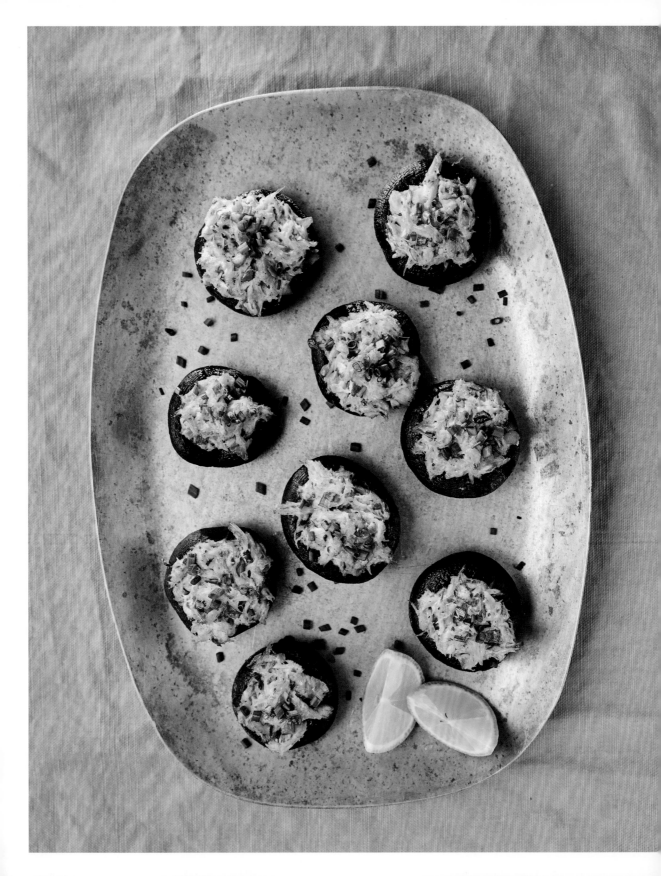

crab-stuffed mushrooms

YIELD 12 SERVINGS

PREP TIME 15 MINUTES

COOK TIME 28 MINUTES

NUT FREE

Two 14-ounce (392 g) containers
stuffing mushrooms (about
24 mushrooms)

1 tablespoon (15 ml) avocado oil

¼ cup (24 g) chopped green onion

¼ teaspoon salt

⅛ teaspoon pepper

Two 6-ounce (170 g) cans crabmeat,
drained

¼ cup (60 ml) mayonnaise,
homemade (page 32) or paleo
store-bought

1 tablespoon (15 ml) lemon juice

½ teaspoon garlic powder

The ultimate appetizer! These tender mushrooms are stuffed with a tasty crabmeat filling. They are easy and elegant.

1. Preheat the oven to 350°F (180°C or gas mark 4).

2. Remove the stems from mushrooms and place them on a cutting board. Clean the mushrooms with a damp cloth or paper towel. Place them in a 13 by 9-inch (33 by 23 cm) pan.

3. Chop the mushroom stems and place them in a large skillet with the avocado oil, green onion, salt, and pepper. Cook for 5 minutes over medium heat.

4. While the mushroom mixture is cooking, place the crab in a medium-size bowl. Add the cooked mushroom mixture, mayo, lemon juice, and garlic powder and stir gently to combine but not break up the crabmeat. Scoop the mixture into the stuffing mushrooms.

5. Bake for 20–23 minutes, or until the mushrooms are tender. Serve immediately.

corn-free cornbread

YIELD 9 SERVINGS

PREP TIME 10 MINUTES

COOK TIME 28 MINUTES

¾ cup (84 g) almond flour

¼ cup (30 g) coconut flour

¼ teaspoon salt

½ teaspoon baking soda

3 large eggs, at room temperature

¼ cup (60 ml) melted ghee

3 tablespoons (44 ml) honey

¼ cup (60 ml) almond milk

It's amazing how much this cornbread tastes like the traditional version even though it doesn't use cornmeal. The almond flour and coconut flour mixture gives it that classic texture, and the honey gives it just the right amount of sweetness.

1. Preheat the oven to 350°F (180°C or gas mark 4). Line a 9 by 9-inch (23 by 23 cm) pan with parchment paper or grease well with coconut oil.

2. Combine the almond flour, coconut flour, salt, and baking soda in a large bowl. Mix well.

3. Add the eggs, ghee, honey, and almond milk and stir to combine.

4. Pour the mixture into the prepared pan and spread evenly. Bake for 25–28 minutes, or until the edges are golden brown. Serve warm. This is great with chili or soup.

5. Store leftovers, covered, at room temperature for up to 2 days or longer in the refrigerator.

scotch eggs

YIELD 6 EGGS

PREP TIME 10 MINUTES

COOK TIME 23 MINUTES

low LOW FODMAP IF HOMEMADE SAUSAGE IS USED, NUT FREE

6 hard-boiled eggs

1 pound (454 g) breakfast sausage, homemade (page 54) or sugar-free store-bought

This recipe makes perfectly cooked hard-boiled eggs wrapped in sausage. They are good warm or cold and are great for on the go!

Quick tip: I like to cook the eggs in the pressure cooker. Place them in the bottom with 1 cup (240 ml) of water and cook on High for 4 minutes. Do a quick release and place the eggs in a bowl of cold water for 3 minutes. Then they are ready to peel and be used.

1. Preheat the oven to 350°F (180°C or gas mark 4). Line a baking sheet with parchment paper.

2. Peel the eggs and pat dry with a paper towel. Divide the sausage mixture into 6 equal portions, about ¼ cup (75 g) each. Roll a portion into a ball with your hands and then press it flat. Place an egg in the center of the sausage and form the meat around it. Squeeze the meat so it is packed on tightly. Place on the prepared baking sheet.

3. Repeat with the remaining eggs and sausage. Bake for 20–23 minutes, or until the meat is golden brown. Serve warm.

4. Store leftovers, covered, in the refrigerator for up to 6 days.

cheese dipping sauce

YIELD 3 CUPS (710 ML)

PREP TIME 10 MINUTES

COOK TIME 20 MINUTES

EGG FREE, **low** LOW FODMAP,
NUT FREE

1½ cups (192 g) chopped carrots
(about 2 medium carrots)

2 cups (266 g) chopped potatoes
(about 3 small russet potatoes)

1 teaspoon salt, divided

1 tablespoon (15 ml) garlic-infused
olive oil

2 tablespoons (30 ml) lemon juice

2 tablespoons (30 g) ghee

¼ teaspoon ground black pepper

This dip is so smooth, it has the same consistency as melted cheese sauce. Grab some veggies, grain-free tortilla chips, or crackers and dig in!

1. Place the carrots, potatoes, and ½ teaspoon of the salt in a large stockpot. Cover with water, cover the pot, and bring to a boil over high heat. Reduce the heat to medium and cook for about 15 minutes, or until the carrots and potatoes are tender.

2. Drain and transfer the vegetables to a high-powdered blender.

3. Add the olive oil, lemon juice, ghee, pepper, and remaining ½ teaspoon salt. Blend on high speed until smooth.

4. Serve as a dip with crackers, veggies, or chips. Or store leftovers, covered, in the refrigerator for up to a week. It will thicken as it cools; rewarm it if you want it thinner.

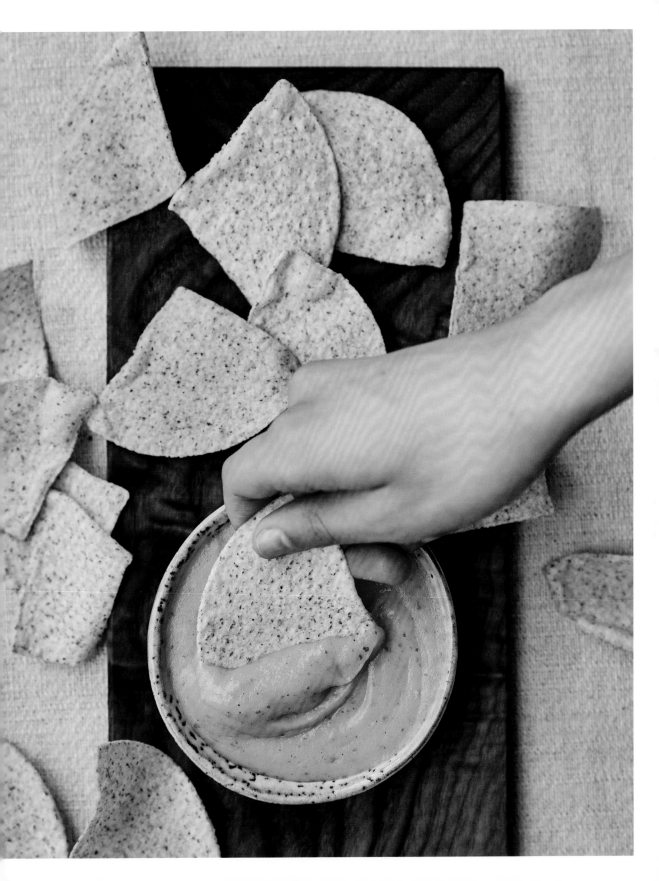

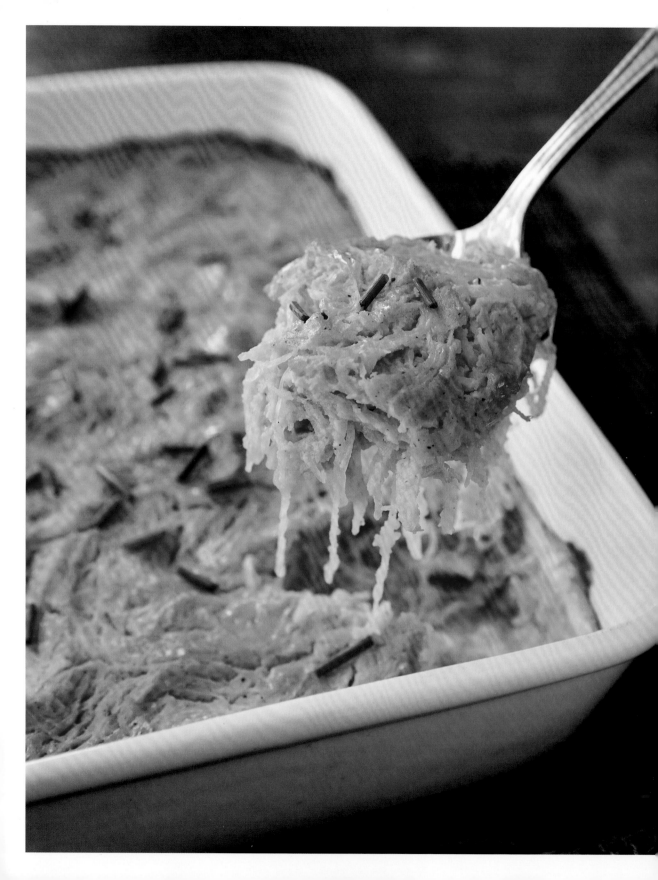

baked mac and cheese

YIELD 6-8 SERVINGS

PREP TIME 20 MINUTES

COOK TIME 50 MINUTES

low LOW FODMAP, NUT FREE IF COCONUT MILK IS USED INSTEAD OF ALMOND MILK

(IF YOU DON'T NEED LOW FODMAP, YOU MAY USE ALL GHEE IN PLACE OF THE OIL AND GHEE COMBINATION AND ADD 1 TEASPOON GARLIC POWDER.)

SAUCE

3 cups (413 g) chopped butternut squash, 1-inch (3 cm) cubes

½ teaspoon salt

¾ cup (180 ml) almond milk

1 teaspoon garlic-infused olive oil

2 tablespoons (30 g) ghee

2 tablespoons (6 g) chopped chives

1 tablespoon (15 ml) lemon juice

¼ teaspoon ground black pepper

½ teaspoon paprika

1 teaspoon yellow mustard

NOODLES

1 recipe Spaghetti Squash (page 37)

2 large eggs, lightly beaten

Creating a grain-free, dairy-free version of macaroni and cheese was a challenge, but I was determined to have one that would not disappoint. This took a few tries to get it just right, and I know you will love it. It's creamy and rich, and will satisfy that craving for the traditional side. Spaghetti squash noodles are the "macaroni" and the cheese sauce is made with a veggie, but the combination is a cozy, luscious dish. The butternut squash is a little sweeter than cheese, which is why the lemon juice is needed. It adds the classic "tang" of cheese while balancing the sweetness.

1. Preheat the oven to 375°F (190°C or gas mark 5). Line a 13 by 9-inch (33 by 23 cm) pan with parchment paper or grease well with coconut oil.

2. Make the sauce: Place the butternut squash and salt in a large stockpot and cover with water. Bring to a boil, covered, over high heat. Reduce the heat to medium-low and cook for about 10 minutes, or until the squash is tender.

3. Strain and transfer the squash to a high-powdered blender. Add the almond milk, olive oil, ghee, chives, lemon juice, pepper, paprika, and mustard. Blend until smooth.

4. Make the noodles: Place the spaghetti squash noodles in a large bowl. Cut the noodles into strips 2–3 inches (5–8 cm) long with clean kitchen scissors. Pour the butternut squash sauce on top of the spaghetti squash. Add the eggs and mix well, until all the noodles are covered.

5. Pour into the prepared pan and bake for 35–40 minutes, or until the top is golden brown. Serve immediately. It's best scooped with a spoon, as it doesn't cut well.

6. Store leftovers, covered, in the refrigerator for up to a week.

classic deviled eggs

YIELD 12 SERVINGS

PREP TIME 10 MINUTES

COOK TIME N/A

low LOW FODMAP, NUT FREE

6 large hard-boiled eggs (see page 69 for a pressure cooker option)

¼ cup (60 ml) mayonnaise, homemade (page 32) or paleo store-bought

1 teaspoon Dijon-style mustard

⅛ teaspoon salt

⅛ teaspoon ground black pepper

These iconic appetizers are perfect for any holiday party or other gathering. No potluck buffet is complete without them! Just a few simple ingredients combine to make a creamy filling for the egg whites. The secret here is to break out your whisk instead of using a fork. A whisk really breaks up the egg yolk chunks and makes the filling smooth and irresistible.

1. Peel the eggs and cut in half lengthwise. Remove the yolks and place them in a medium-size bowl. Arrange the egg whites on a plate (slicing off a tiny piece from the bottom makes them sit up straight).

2. Add the mayonnaise, mustard, salt, and pepper to the egg yolks and whisk to combine.

3. Spoon the filling evenly into each egg white. Serve immediately or chill before serving.

4. Store leftovers, covered, in the refrigerator for up to 5 days.

spinach artichoke dip

YIELD 8-10 SERVINGS

PREP TIME 15 MINUTES

COOK TIME 25 MINUTES

low LOW FODMAP, NUT FREE

(IF YOU DON'T NEED LOW FODMAP, REPLACE THE GARLIC-INFUSED OLIVE OIL WITH 1 TEASPOON GARLIC POWDER AND JUST USE MORE AVOCADO OIL.)

1 tablespoon (15 ml) avocado oil

10 ounces (283 g) baby spinach, chopped

One 14-ounce (392 g) can artichoke hearts, drained and chopped

½ teaspoon salt

2 tablespoons (30 ml) garlic-infused olive oil

⅔ cup (158 ml) mayonnaise, homemade (page 32) or paleo store-bought

2 tablespoons (30 ml) lemon juice

½ teaspoon ground black pepper

2 teaspoons (7 g) arrowroot powder

This dip is rich, creamy, and full of flavor. Baked until warm and bubbly, it's always a crowd-pleaser. And it's not hard to make!

1. Preheat the oven to 350°F (180°C or gas mark 4). Grease a 7½ by 6-inch (19 by 15 cm) baking pan (or other small ovenproof dish) with coconut oil.

2. Heat the avocado oil in a large skillet over medium heat. Add the spinach and cook for about 3 minutes, or until the spinach is wilted. Add the chopped artichokes, salt, olive oil, mayonnaise, lemon juice, and pepper and mix well. Sprinkle in the arrowroot powder and cook for about 2 minutes, or until thickened.

3. Pour into the prepared dish and bake for 20 minutes, or until bubbly and golden brown. Serve warm with veggies or grain-free crackers.

4. Store leftovers, covered, in the refrigerator for up to 5 days.

sausage balls

YIELD 21 BALLS

PREP TIME 5 MINUTES

COOK TIME 20 MINUTES

EGG FREE

1 pound (454 g) breakfast sausage, homemade (page 54) or sugar-free store bought

1 cup (112 g) almond flour

1 teaspoon baking soda

This classic appetizer is made over to be gluten and dairy free. The baking soda in the sausage balls gives them a bubbly outside that is slightly crispy. Use any sausage you like for the spice level you desire.

1. Preheat the oven to 400°F (200°C or gas mark 6). Line a baking sheet with parchment paper.

2. Combine the sausage, almond flour, and baking soda in a large bowl. With your hands, scoop with a spoon into 1-inch (3 cm) balls, making about 21.

3. Arrange the balls on the prepared baking sheet and bake for 18–20 minutes, or until browned and crispy. Serve immediately.

4. Store leftovers, covered, in the refrigerator for up to 6 days.

cheese ball

YIELD 6-8 SERVINGS

PREP TIME 15 MINUTES (PLUS 6 HOURS TO SOAK CASHEWS)

COOK TIME N/A

EGG FREE

2 cups (224 g) raw cashews

½ teaspoon salt

2 tablespoons (30 ml) lemon juice

1 teaspoon garlic powder

2-3 tablespoons (30-45 ml) water

2 teaspoons chopped chives

I used to be known for the cheese balls that I would bring to family gatherings. Unfortunately, they were always made with cream cheese and seasoning packets. But I knew there would definitely be a way to make them dairy free and with all real seasonings. Cashews replace the cheese in this dairy-free cheese ball. The texture and taste are spot-on to a real cheese ball. It's creamy, tangy, and so scrumptious. I served this at my family Christmas dinner, and everyone went wild for it.

1. In a medium-size bowl, soak the cashews in filtered water for 6 hours.

2. Drain, rinse, and transfer the cashews to a high-powdered blender. Add the salt, lemon juice, garlic powder, and 2 table-spoons (30 ml) water. Blend slowly, stopping and scraping down the sides as needed. Add an extra 1 tablespoon (15 ml) water if needed, but be patient. It takes about 5 minutes for the mixture to become smooth.

3. Place a piece of plastic wrap in a bowl and scoop the mixture into it. Wrap the plastic wrap around the mixture, shaping it into a ball. Twist closed and place in the refrigerator to chill.

4. Unwrap the cheese ball, place it on a plate, and serve it with veggies or grain-free crackers.

5. Store leftovers, covered, in the refrigerator for up to 10 days.

Recipes

Chapter 6

---

mains: chicken, turkey, and pork

Chicken, turkey, and pork are dinnertime go-tos. They can
sometimes be dry and flavorless, but not these recipes!
These are some of my favorites in this book. You will
find cozy casseroles, flavorful meatballs, and decadent
skillet meals.

bourbon chicken

YIELD 4–6 SERVINGS

PREP TIME 5 MINUTES

COOK TIME 27 MINUTES

NUT FREE, EGG FREE

This used to be my favorite dish to buy from the mall food court. This remake, named after the famed street in New Orleans, has much less sugar, but it still has all the flavor! It's delicious served with zucchini noodles or cauliflower rice.

1 tablespoon (15 ml) garlic-infused olive oil

2 pounds (907 g) boneless skinless chicken breasts, cut into 1-inch (3 cm) pieces

½ teaspoon salt

¼ teaspoon ground black pepper

¼ cup (60 ml) apple juice

2 tablespoons (30 ml) ketchup, homemade (page 33) or paleo store-bought (I like Primal Kitchen)

⅓ cup (80 ml) coconut aminos

½ cup (120 ml) water

¼ teaspoon ground ginger

1 tablespoon (10 g) arrowroot powder/starch

1. Heat the olive oil in a large skillet over medium heat. Add the chicken, salt, and pepper. Cook, stirring regularly, for 5 minutes. The chicken will not be fully cooked at this point. Transfer to a plate.

2. Add the apple juice, ketchup, coconut aminos, water, and ginger. Cook for 10 minutes, or until slightly reduced. Add the arrowroot powder, whisk to combine, and stir with a spoon for about 2 minutes, or until the sauce thickens. Add the chicken back in and cook for 10 minutes, or until the chicken is cooked through. Serve warm.

3. Store leftovers, covered, in the refrigerator for up to 6 days.

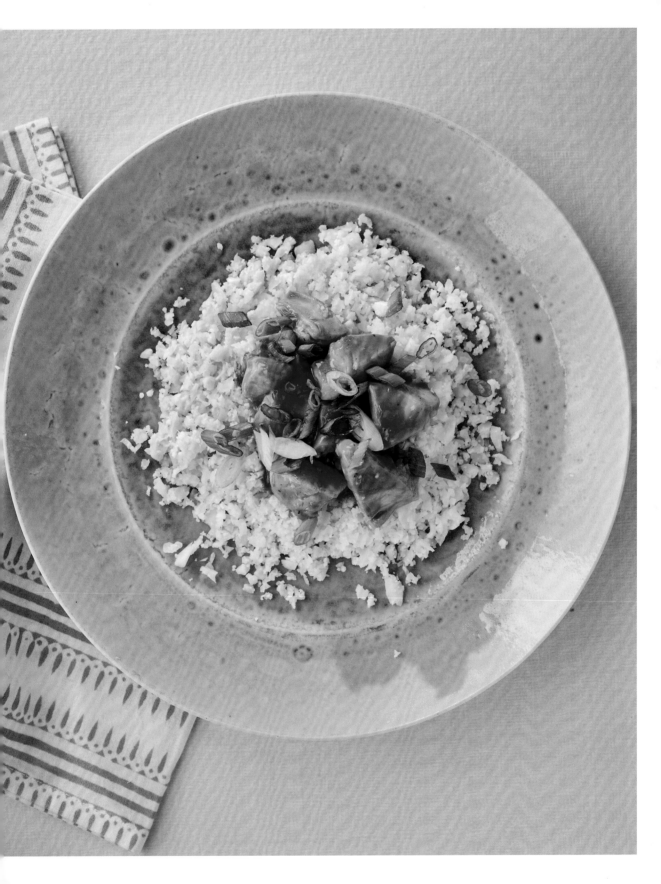

southwest chicken meatballs

YIELD 16 MEATBALLS

PREP TIME 15 MINUTES

COOK TIME 18 MINUTES

low LOW FODMAP, EGG FREE AND NUT FREE IF YOU LEAVE THE EGG AND ALMOND FLOUR OUT AND USE 1 TABLESPOON (1 G) GELATIN IN THE MEATBALLS

(IF YOU DON'T NEED LOW FODMAP, YOU MAY USE 1 TEASPOON GARLIC POWDER IN PLACE OF THE GARLIC-INFUSED OLIVE OIL.)

MEATBALLS

1 pound (454 g) ground turkey

¼ cup (4 g) chopped cilantro

¼ cup (24 g) chopped green onion

1 tablespoon (15 ml) garlic-infused olive oil

3 tablespoons (31 g) finely diced red bell pepper

1 teaspoon salt

¼ teaspoon ground black pepper

½ teaspoon ground cumin

1 large egg

¼ cup (28 g) almond flour

SAUCE

One 13.5-ounce (378 ml) can full-fat coconut milk

½ cup (8 g) chopped cilantro

¼ cup (24 g) chopped green onion

2 tablespoons (30 ml) garlic-infused olive oil

⅛ teaspoon ground black pepper

⅛ teaspoon salt

Fresh cilantro and green onion add so much flavor to these meatballs! They are served with a creamy sauce, and the combination is divine.

1. Preheat the oven to 400°F (200°C or gas mark 6). Line a baking sheet with parchment paper.

2. Make the meatballs: Place the turkey in a large bowl. Add the cilantro, green onion, olive oil, bell pepper, salt, pepper, cumin, egg, and almond flour. Mix well with a wooden spoon, until all the ingredients are distributed evenly.

3. With your hands, scoop into heaping 1-tablespoon (15 g) balls and arrange on the prepared baking sheet.

4. Bake for 16–18 minutes.

5. While the meatballs bake, make the sauce: Place the coconut milk, cilantro, green onion, olive oil, pepper, and salt in a blender and blend on high speed until smooth.

6. Serve the meatballs with the sauce. Store leftovers, covered, in the refrigerator for up to 6 days.

chicken curry waffles

YIELD 4 SERVINGS

PREP TIME 5 MINUTES

COOK TIME 8 MINUTES

low LOW FODMAP

(IF YOU DON'T NEED LOW FODMAP, YOU MAY USE ½ TEASPOON GARLIC POWDER IN PLACE OF THE OIL.)

Two 5-ounce (142 g) cans organic chicken with no additives, drained

1 large egg

1 tablespoon (7 g) curry powder

½ teaspoon ground ginger

1 tablespoon (15 ml) garlic-infused olive oil

¼ cup (28 g) almond flour

¼ teaspoon ground black pepper

¼ cup (60 ml) full-fat coconut milk

Ghee, for serving (optional)

I have a few versions of savory waffles on my website that get a lot of love, so I knew I wanted to include one here. These use canned chicken, and the curry powder gives them lots of flavor. They are the best quick lunch.

1. Warm up the waffle maker while the mixture is being mixed.

2. Combine the chicken, egg, curry powder, ginger, olive oil, almond flour, pepper, and coconut milk in a large bowl. Mix until everything is well combined. Divide the mixture into 4 portions. Shape each portion into a ball and place it on a plate to be ready to put in the waffle maker.

3. Once the waffle maker is ready, place the patties on it, close it, and cook for 4 minutes.

4. Carefully remove the waffles, transferring to a plate. Repeat as necessary with the remaining batter. (I have a smaller waffle maker, so I cook 2 at a time.) Serve immediately with a little ghee on top, if desired.

5. Store leftovers, covered, in the refrigerator for up to 6 days.

chicken bacon ranch meatloaf

YIELD 8 SERVINGS

PREP TIME 10 MINUTES

COOK TIME 1 HOUR 10 MINUTES

`low` LOW FODMAP IF HOMEMADE RANCH DRESSING IS USED

2 pounds (907 g) ground chicken or turkey

2 large eggs

½ cup (56 g) almond flour

1 cup (240 ml) ranch dressing, homemade (page 36) or paleo store-bought, divided

⅓ cup (32 g) chopped green onion

1½ teaspoons salt

10 pieces bacon, cooked and crumbled

Crispy bacon, cool ranch dressing, and ground chicken (or turkey) make this meatloaf super flavorful! It's great the day you make it and even better the next day.

1. Preheat the oven to 375°F (190°C or gas mark 5). Line a baking sheet with parchment paper.

2. Combine the chicken, eggs, almond flour, ½ cup (120 ml) of the ranch dressing, green onion, salt, and bacon in a large bowl. Mix well, until all the ingredients are well incorporated.

3. Place the mixture onto the baking sheet and form into a 10½ by 6-inch (27 by 15 cm) loaf. Bake for 40 minutes.

4. Top with the remaining ½ cup (120 ml) ranch dressing, spreading it evenly. Bake for 30 more minutes. Slice and serve warm.

5. Store leftovers, covered, in the refrigerator for up to a week.

deviled ham

YIELD 4-6 SERVINGS

PREP TIME 10 MINUTES

COOK TIME N/A

NUT FREE

This savory spread is a fantastic way to use up leftover ham. It's creamy and thick, and great paired with fresh veggies or grain-free crackers.

1 pound (454 g) sugar-free ham

¼ large onion

1 teaspoon yellow mustard

½ cup (120 ml) mayonnaise, homemade (page 32) or paleo store-bought

2 tablespoons (30 g) dill pickle relish

1. Place the ham and onion in a food processor and chop finely. Add the mustard, mayonnaise, and relish and blend until combined. Serve immediately or chill in the refrigerator.

2. Store leftovers, covered, in the refrigerator for up to a week.

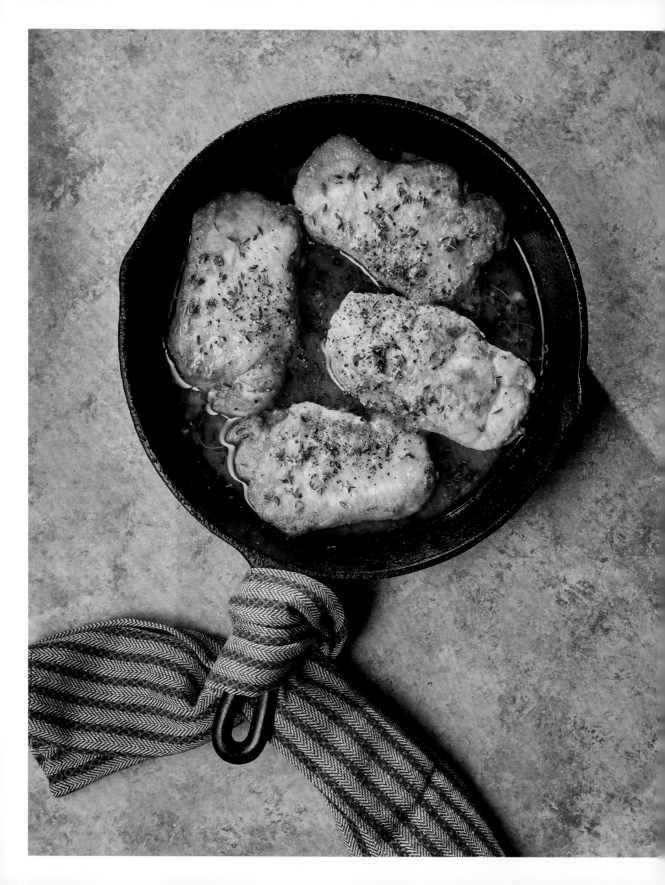

creamy lemon thyme pork chops

YIELD 4 SERVINGS

PREP TIME 5 MINUTES

COOK TIME 25 MINUTES

low LOW FODMAP

(IF YOU DON'T NEED LOW FODMAP, YOU MAY USE AVOCADO OIL AND 1 TEASPOON GARLIC POWDER IN PLACE OF THE GARLIC-INFUSED OLIVE OIL.)

¼ cup (37 g) cassava flour

1 teaspoon salt

¼ teaspoon ground black pepper

4 pork chops, 1 inch (3 cm) thick (about 2 pounds [907 g])

2 tablespoons (30 ml) garlic-infused olive oil

Zest of 1 lemon

⅓ cup (80 ml) lemon juice

1 tablespoon (6 g) chopped fresh thyme

⅓ cup (80 g) ghee

Pork chops can be dry and boring, but not these! They are juicy and have great fresh flavor from the thyme and lemon.

1. Mix the cassava flour, salt, and pepper in a shallow bowl. Dredge the pork chops in the flour mixture, coating all sides. There may be some mixture left over.

2. Heat a large pan over medium heat and add the olive oil. Let it warm for 2 minutes. Add the pork chops and cook for 6 minutes without moving them. Flip and cook for 3 more minutes.

3. Transfer the pork chops to a plate. Add the lemon zest and juice, thyme, and ghee to the pan and cook for 2 minutes, or until a sauce is formed.

4. Add the pork chops back in and cook over low heat for 6–10 minutes, or until they reach 155°F (68°C) on a meat thermometer. Spoon the sauce over the pork chops as they cook.

5. Remove from the oven and serve immediately.

6. Store leftovers, covered, in the refrigerator for up to 6 days.

easy roast chicken

YIELD 4-6 SERVINGS

PREP TIME 10 MINUTES

COOK TIME 1 HOUR 20 MINUTES

EGG FREE, **low** LOW FODMAP, NUT FREE

Here's a simple recipe that results in a juicy roast with crispy skin. It's great served fresh, and then you can use the leftover meat for other meals.

4- to 5-pound (1.8-2.3 kg) whole chicken

2 tablespoons (30 ml) melted ghee

1 tablespoon (15 ml) garlic-infused olive oil

Zest and juice of 1 lemon

1 teaspoon salt

¼ teaspoon ground black pepper

1. Preheat the oven to 375°F (190°C or gas mark 5). Place the chicken in a roasting pan or on a rimmed baking sheet. Remove the giblets from inside the chicken and discard or save for another use.

2. Stir together the ghee, olive oil, lemon zest, and lemon juice in a small bowl. Drizzle over the chicken, making sure it's coated well.

3. Sprinkle with the salt and pepper and bake for 70–80 minutes, or until the meat reaches 165°F (74°C) on a meat thermometer at the thickest part.

4. Let the chicken rest for 10 minutes. Slice the chicken, transfer to a platter, and serve.

5. Store leftovers, covered, in the refrigerator for up to 6 days.

apple pork chops

YIELD 6 SERVINGS

PREP TIME 10 MINUTES

COOK TIME 25 MINUTES

EGG FREE, NUT FREE

PORK CHOPS

6 pork chops (2 pounds [907 g] total)

2 tablespoons (30 ml) melted ghee

2 teaspoons salt

1 teaspoon dried sage

APPLE TOPPING

2 medium apples, cored and sliced

1 tablespoon (15 g) ghee

⅛ teaspoon salt

½ teaspoon ground cinnamon

2 tablespoons (30 ml) water
(optional)

Apple picking or just visiting the local farmers' market is one of my favorite fall activities. It usually results in lots of fresh apples and new ways to enjoy them. Pairing them with perfectly juicy pork chops is delicious. The apples are tender and sweet and add great autumn flavor to the dish. This is a light and flavorful meal that is sure to please.

1. Preheat the oven to 400°F (200°C or gas mark 6). Line a baking sheet with parchment paper.

2. Make the pork chops: Place the pork chops on the prepared baking sheet, brush with the ghee on both sides, and sprinkle with the salt and sage.

3. Bake for 20–25 minutes, or until the pork reaches 145°F (63°C) on a meat thermometer.

4. While the pork chops cook, make the apple topping: Place the apples, ghee, salt, and cinnamon in a large skillet over medium heat and cook for 8–10 minutes. Add the water if needed to prevent sticking during cooking.

5. Transfer the pork chops to a platter and ladle the apples over them to serve.

6. Store leftovers, covered, in the refrigerator for up to 6 days.

pork rind–crusted pork chops

YIELD 2 SERVINGS

PREP TIME 10 MINUTES

COOK TIME 27 MINUTES

EGG FREE, <mark>low</mark> LOW FODMAP,
NUT FREE

(IF YOU DON'T NEED LOW FODMAP,
YOU MAY USE A FLAVORED PORK RIND
IF DESIRED.)

2 tablespoons (30 ml) melted ghee

2 ounces (57 g) plain pork rinds,
blended or crushed until fine (look
for humanely raised pork rinds,
such as Epic or 4505)

½ teaspoon salt

¼ teaspoon ground black pepper

2 pork chops, 1 inch (3 cm) thick
(1 pound [454 g] total)

*If you are looking for a crunchy coated pork chop, this is it! The
pork rinds crisp up so nicely and make the most amazing crust.*

1. Preheat the oven to 400°F (200°C or gas mark 6). Line a
   rimmed baking sheet with parchment paper. Put a wire rack
   on top of the baking sheet. This will help keep the pork chops
   crispy as they cook.

2. Place the melted ghee in a shallow dish and the pork rinds in
   a separate shallow dish along with the salt and pepper. Dip the
   pork chops in the ghee, coating fully, then in the pork rinds.
   Press the pork rinds into the chops to help them stick.

3. Place the pork chops on the wire rack and bake for
   23–27 minutes, or until they reach 145°F (63°C) on a meat
   thermometer.

4. Remove from the oven and serve immediately.

chicken parmesan casserole

YIELD 4–6 SERVINGS

PREP TIME 20 MINUTES

COOK TIME 47 MINUTES

`low` LOW FODMAP IF SENSITIVE MARINARA IS USED (RAO'S IS MY FAVORITE)

(IF YOU DON'T NEED LOW FODMAP, YOU MAY USE YOUR FAVORITE MARINARA SAUCE. YOU MAY USE AVOCADO OIL IN PLACE OF THE GARLIC-INFUSED OLIVE OIL AND ADD 1 TEASPOON GARLIC POWDER.)

CASSEROLE

1 small (2-pound [907 g]) spaghetti squash, cooked and shredded into noodles (see page 37)

1 large egg

1 teaspoon Italian seasoning

¾ teaspoon salt, divided

1¼ cups (296 ml) marinara sauce

1 tablespoon (15 ml) garlic-infused olive oil

1 pound (454 g) boneless skinless chicken breasts, cut into ½-inch (1 cm) chunks

TOPPING

1 cup (112 g) almond flour

1 tablespoon (8 g) coconut flour

½ teaspoon salt

1 teaspoon Italian seasoning

2 tablespoons (30 ml) melted ghee

This casserole was a delightful accident. I was trying to create a classic chicken Parmesan, and it wasn't turning out how I wanted. I decided to turn it into a casserole with a crumble topping, and it exceeded my expectations. The topping is reminiscent of Parmesan cheese! This is a comforting dish that is beyond delicious.

1. Preheat the oven to 350°F (180°C or gas mark 4). Line a 9 by 9-inch (23 by 23 cm) pan with parchment paper or grease well with coconut oil.

2. Make the casserole: Place the spaghetti squash in a large bowl. Add the egg, Italian seasoning, and ¼ teaspoon of the salt and mix well. Place in the bottom of the prepared pan.

3. Top with the marinara sauce.

4. Heat the olive oil in a large skillet over medium heat. Add the chicken and remaining ½ teaspoon salt and cook for 5–7 minutes. It will not be fully cooked at this point. Arrange the chicken on top of the marinara.

5. Make the topping: Combine the almond flour, coconut flour, salt, Italian seasoning, and ghee in a small bowl. Mix until crumbly. Sprinkle the topping over the chicken.

6. Bake for 40 minutes, or until golden brown.

7. Remove from the oven and serve immediately.

8. Store leftovers, covered, in the refrigerator for up to 6 days.

pecan-crusted chicken tenders

YIELD 4 SERVINGS

PREP TIME 10 MINUTES

COOK TIME 17 MINUTES

EGG FREE, **low** LOW FODMAP

(IF YOU DON'T NEED LOW FODMAP, YOU MAY USE ALL GHEE INSTEAD OF THE GHEE AND OIL MIXTURE, AND ADD ½ TEASPOON GARLIC POWDER TO THE PECAN MIXTURE.)

1¼ cups (140 g) finely chopped raw pecans

1 teaspoon salt

¼ teaspoon ground black pepper

1 teaspoon dried chives

1 tablespoon (15 ml) melted ghee

1 tablespoon (15 ml) garlic-infused olive oil

1–1¼ pounds (454–567 kg) chicken tenders or breasts cut into strips

This tender chicken is coated in crunchy pecans that are baked to perfection. These will be loved by the whole family!

1. Preheat the oven to 400°F (200°C or gas mark 6). Line a baking sheet with parchment paper and then place a wire rack on top. This will help the chicken stay crispy.

2. Place the pecans in a shallow dish and add the salt, pepper, and chives. Mix well.

3. In a separate shallow dish, combine the melted ghee and olive oil.

4. Dip the chicken pieces into the ghee mixture and then into the pecan mixture. Press the pecans onto the chicken so they adhere. Place on the wire rack on the prepared baking sheet.

5. Repeat with the remaining chicken.

6. Bake for 14–17 minutes, or until the coating is crisp and golden.

7. Remove from the oven and serve immediately. They are great by themselves but you can also use paleo ranch dressing (page 36) as a dip.

8. Store leftovers, covered, in the refrigerator for up to 6 days.

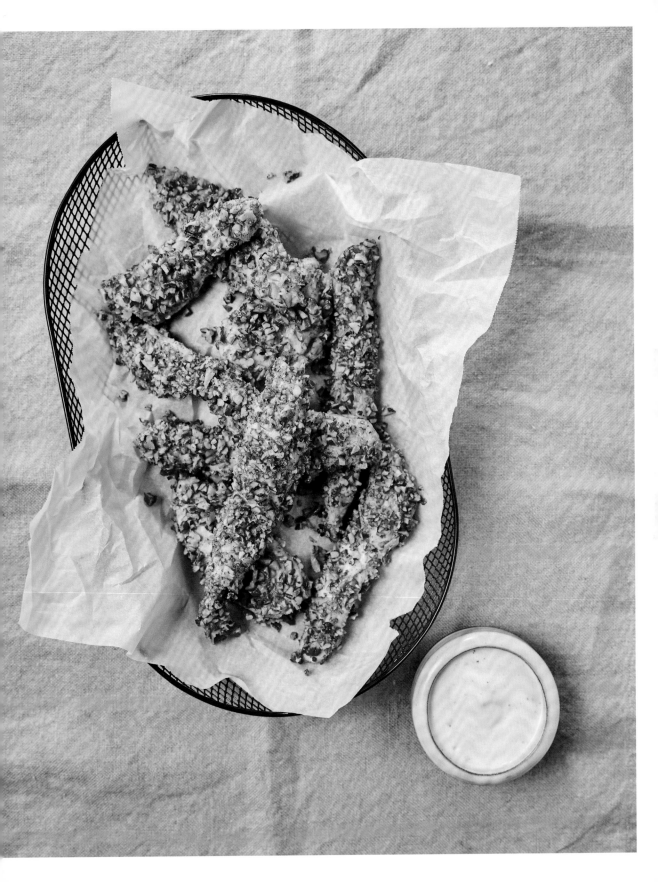

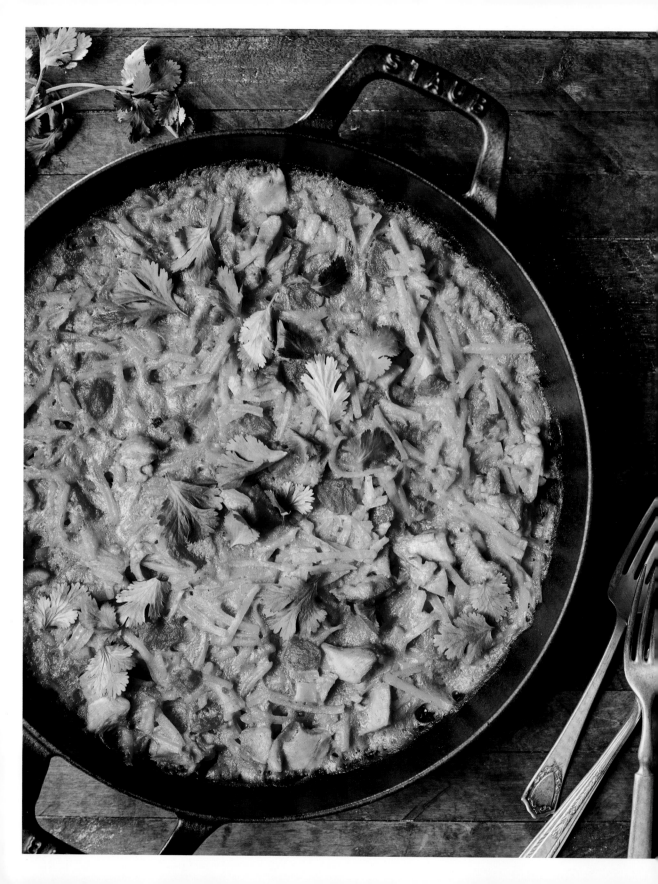

chicken curry casserole

YIELD 4–6 SERVINGS

PREP TIME 20 MINUTES

COOK TIME 50 MINUTES

EGG FREE, NUT FREE,
`low` LOW FODMAP IF CURRY POWDER
DOESN'T HAVE GARLIC OR ONION
(I USE FRONTIER CO-OP BRAND.)

(IF YOU DON'T NEED LOW FODMAP,
YOU MAY USE 2 FRESH CLOVES GARLIC,
MINCED, IN PLACE OF THE GARLIC-
INFUSED OIL AND USE ANY CURRY
YOU PREFER.)

One 14.5-ounce (411 g) can diced
tomatoes

One 13.5-ounce (378 ml) can full-fat
coconut milk

1 tablespoon (15 ml) garlic-infused
olive oil

1½ teaspoons (9 g) salt

1½ tablespoons (11 g) curry powder

1 teaspoon ground ginger

1½ pounds (680 g) boneless skinless
chicken thighs

1 pound (454 g) frozen hash browns
(no need to thaw first)

This is a super simple curry combined with shredded potatoes to make a comforting casserole. My four-year-old daughter loves curry, which means I make it often. Finding a new way to enjoy it was nice, and she loves this dish. It's not spicy, making it very kid-friendly.

1. Preheat the oven to 350°F (180°C or gas mark 4). Line a 9 by 9-inch (23 by 23 cm) pan with parchment paper.

2. Combine the tomatoes, coconut milk, olive oil, salt, curry powder, and ginger in a saucepan. Put the chicken thighs in, making sure they are fully covered. Place the saucepan over medium heat and bring the mixture to a simmer, about 5 minutes. Decrease the heat to medium-low, cover, and cook, stirring regularly, for 13 minutes.

3. Transfer the chicken to a cutting board and leave the sauce to keep cooking. Chop the chicken into bite-size pieces and place it back in the pan. Turn off the heat.

4. Place the hash browns in a large bowl and add to the chicken. Mix well and pour into the prepared pan. Bake for 40–50 minutes.

5. Remove from the oven and serve immediately.

6. Store leftovers, covered, in the refrigerator for up to 6 days.

buffalo chicken casserole

YIELD 6-8 SERVINGS

PREP TIME 45 MINUTES

COOK TIME 35 MINUTES

NUT FREE, EGG FREE IF YOU LEAVE
OUT THE EGGS (THEY HELP HOLD
THE CASSEROLE TOGETHER, BUT CAN
BE LEFT OUT IF THERE IS AN ALLERGY
OR SENSITIVITY.)

This is the most popular casserole on my website, made by hundreds of people, and definitely deserving of a spot here! This dish is packed with veggies and flavor while still being total comfort food.

Tip: Start with ½ cup (120 ml) of the hot sauce and increase the amount if you like. This casserole is very spicy if you use the full cup, but a lot of people love it that way.

1 large spaghetti squash

1 tablespoon (15 ml) avocado oil

1 large onion, diced

1 cup (128 g) diced carrots
(2-3 medium carrots)

2 pounds (907 g) cooked chicken

½-1 cup (120-240 ml) Frank's
RedHot

¼ cup (60 ml) ranch dressing,
homemade (page 36) or paleo
store-bought, plus extra for serving
(optional)

1 teaspoon garlic powder

¼ teaspoon salt

¼ teaspoon ground black pepper

3 large eggs, lightly beaten

1. Preheat the oven to 400°F (200°C or gas mark 6). Line a baking sheet with parchment paper. Line a 13 by 9-inch (33 by 23 cm) pan with parchment paper.

2. Cut the squash in half, remove the seeds, place cut side down on the prepared baking sheet, and bake for 35–45 minutes, or until tender.

3. While the squash is cooking, heat the oil in a large skillet over medium heat. Add the onion and carrots and sauté for 5–7 minutes, or until softened and mostly cooked through.

4. Shred the squash with a fork and transfer it to a large bowl. Press the liquid out with a clean towel. It doesn't have to be super dry, but this helps keep the casserole from getting too watery.

5. Add the onion mixture, chicken, hot sauce, ranch dressing (if using), garlic powder, salt, and pepper to the bowl. Stir well.

6. Add the eggs, mix well, and pour the mixture into the prepared pan.

7. Bake for 30–35 minutes, or until the top is golden brown and bubbly. Serve with additional ranch dressing (if using) if desired.

8. Store leftovers, covered, in the refrigerator for up to 6 days.

creamy chicken and broccoli casserole

YIELD 6–8 SERVINGS

PREP TIME 20 MINUTES

COOK TIME 40 MINUTES

EGG FREE, **low** LOW FODMAP,
NUT FREE IF COCONUT MILK IS USED
IN PLACE OF ALMOND MILK

5 cups (425 g) broccoli florets

1 tablespoon (15 ml) avocado oil

¼ teaspoon salt

4 large zucchini, shredded

1 bunch green onions, chopped
(about ½ cup [48 g])

2 pounds (907 g) boneless skinless
chicken breasts

SAUCE

3 tablespoons (21 g) cassava flour

2 tablespoons (30 g) ghee

1 tablespoon (15 ml) garlic-infused
olive oil

3 cups (710 ml) almond milk

1 teaspoon salt

½ teaspoon ground black pepper

*This dish is packed with veggies and is incredibly tasty. It features
tender chicken, a creamy sauce, and perfectly cooked broccoli.*

1. Preheat the oven to 425°F (220°C or gas mark 7). Line a baking
   sheet with parchment paper. Grease a 13 by 9-inch (33 by 23 cm)
   pan well with coconut oil.

2. Place the broccoli on the prepared baking sheet, drizzle
   with the oil, and sprinkle with the salt. Toss to coat. Bake for
   10 minutes.

3. Place the shredded zucchini, green onions, and raw chicken
   in a large bowl.

4. Make the sauce while the broccoli bakes: Place the cassava
   flour, ghee, and olive oil in a large skillet over medium heat.
   Whisk to combine. Add the almond milk, salt, and pepper and
   heat for about 5 minutes, or until thickened. Pour over the
   zucchini and chicken.

5. When the broccoli is done, lower the oven temperature to
   375°F (190°C or gas mark 5) and add the broccoli to the bowl
   with the other ingredients, stir to combine, and pour the
   mixture into the prepared pan. Bake for 35–40 minutes, or
   until golden brown.

6. If the casserole is too liquidy, scoop out the excess water with
   a spoon. Serve warm.

7. Store leftovers, covered, in the refrigerator for up to 6 days.

cabbage sausage skillet

YIELD 6 SERVINGS

PREP TIME 15 MINUTES

COOK TIME 30 MINUTES

EGG FREE, NUT FREE

CABBAGE AND SAUSAGE

1 tablespoon (15 ml) avocado oil

12 ounces (340 g) sugar-free kielbasa (such as Pederson's Farms), sliced into ½-inch (1 cm) slices

1 onion, diced

3 cloves garlic, minced

½ teaspoon salt

1 large head cabbage (about 3 pounds [1.4 kg]), chopped

SAUCE

2 tablespoons (30 g) spicy brown mustard

1 tablespoon (15 ml) apple cider vinegar

¼ cup (60 ml) olive oil

¼ teaspoon ground black pepper

½ teaspoon garlic powder

This simple meal comes together quickly. It is flavorful and filling, and the sauce pairs perfectly with the cabbage and sausage.

1. Heat the avocado oil in a large skillet over medium heat. Add the sausage and cook, stirring regularly, for 5 minutes. Add the onion, garlic, and salt and cook, stirring regularly, for 5 more minutes.

2. Add the cabbage, in portions if the pan isn't big enough, and cook, stirring regularly, for 15–20 minutes, or until the cabbage is tender.

3. While the cabbage is cooking, make the sauce: Combine the mustard, vinegar, olive oil, pepper, and garlic powder in a small bowl. Mix well.

4. Turn off the heat and stir the sauce into the cabbage mixture. Serve immediately.

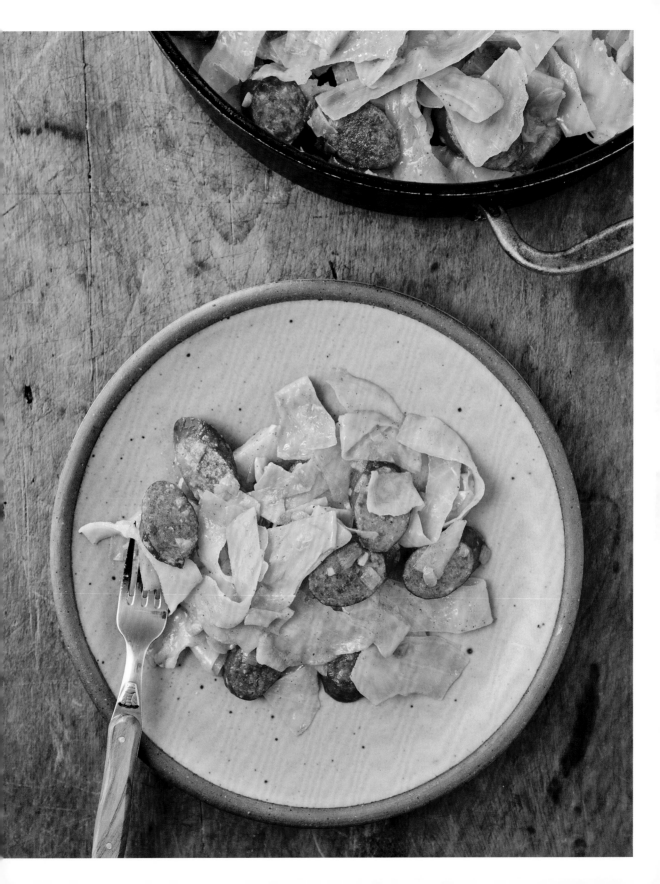

pizza lasagna

YIELD 6 SERVINGS

PREP TIME 21 MINUTES

COOK TIME 65 MINUTES

EGG FREE, NUT FREE

POTATOES

1½ pounds (680 g) white potatoes, sliced

1 tablespoon (15 ml) avocado oil

¼ teaspoon salt

MEAT MIXTURE

1 tablespoon (15 ml) avocado oil

8 ounces (227 g) mushrooms, chopped

1 bell pepper, cored and diced

1 small sweet onion, diced

1 teaspoon garlic powder

¼ teaspoon salt

1 pound (454 g) Italian sausage

1 tablespoon (6 g) dried oregano

One 24-ounce (680 g) jar sugar-free marinara sauce

3 ounces (85 g) pepperoni, diced

With its layers of tender potatoes and a meat mixture that has all the flavors of pizza, this is a must-make for any pizza lover!

1. Preheat the oven to 400°F (200°C or gas mark 6). Line a baking sheet with parchment paper. Line a 9 by 9-inch (23 by 23 cm) pan with parchment paper.

2. Spread the sliced potatoes on the prepared baking sheet, drizzle with the oil, sprinkle with the salt, and toss to evenly coat. They may not fit in an even layer, but that's okay because they're just getting partially cooked. Bake for 15 minutes.

3. While the potatoes bake, make the meat mixture: Heat the avocado oil in a large skillet over medium heat. Add the mushrooms, bell pepper, onion, garlic powder, and salt and cook for 5–8 minutes, or until the veggies start to soften. Add the sausage and oregano and cook for about 8 minutes, or until the sausage is cooked through. Drain the grease if there is a lot. Add the marinara sauce and pepperoni and cook for 5 minutes. Turn off the heat.

4. When the potatoes are ready, decrease the oven temperature to 375°F (190°C or gas mark 5).

5. Place 1½ cups (360 g) of the meat mixture in the bottom of the prepared pan. Top with one-fourth of the potatoes, making an even layer. Repeat with the meat, potatoes, meat, potatoes, meat, and ending with the potatoes.

6. Cover the pan with foil and bake for 30 minutes. Remove the foil and bake for 20 more minutes, or until the top is lightly browned.

7. Remove from the oven, slice, and serve immediately.

8. Store leftovers, covered, in the refrigerator for up to 6 days.

creamy cajun chicken over zucchini noodles

YIELD 6-8 SERVINGS

PREP TIME 15 MINUTES

COOK TIME 20 MINUTES

EGG FREE, NUT FREE

2 tablespoons (30 ml) avocado oil

2 bell peppers, cored and diced

1 large onion, diced

6 boneless skinless chicken thighs, cut into ½-inch (1 cm) pieces

12 ounces (340 g) andouille sausage (I use Pederson's), sliced into ½-inch (1 cm) pieces

One 13.5-ounce (378 ml) can full-fat coconut milk

3 or 4 medium zucchini, spiralized

Chicken thighs and sausage combine with a zesty sauce for one incredible meal. It's a little smoky and has just a little spice.

1. Heat the avocado oil in a large skillet over medium heat. Add the bell peppers and onion and cook for 5–7 minutes, or until the veggies start to get tender.

2. Add the chicken thighs and cook for 5 minutes. Add the sausage and cook for 3 minutes.

3. Add the coconut milk and cook for 5 minutes, or until warmed. Serve over the zucchini noodles or stir the zucchini noodles into the sauce.

4. Store leftovers, covered, in the refrigerator for up to 6 days.

egg roll in a bowl

YIELD 6-8 SERVINGS

PREP TIME 15 MINUTES

COOK TIME 1 HOUR, 5 MINUTES

EGG FREE, NUT FREE

A deconstructed egg roll made healthier and easier! I love this dish because it's packed with veggies, easy to make, and full of flavor. It makes a big batch, and leftovers are just as good—or better! It's topped with a sweet and sour sauce, just like the original.

EGG ROLL IN A BOWL

2 tablespoons (26 g) coconut oil

2 tablespoons (30 ml) sesame oil

1 large head cabbage, sliced

1 large onion, sliced

1 cup (128 g) chopped carrot
(about 1 medium carrot)

1-inch (3 cm) piece fresh ginger,
peeled and grated

3 cloves garlic, grated or minced

¼ cup (60 ml) coconut aminos

1½ pounds (680 g) ground pork
or chicken

SWEET AND SOUR SAUCE

1 tablespoon (15 ml) avocado oil

1 large onion, diced

3 cloves garlic, minced

½ teaspoon salt

¼ teaspoon ground black pepper

One 8-oz (227 g) can crushed
pineapple in juice, not syrup

¼ cup (66 g) tomato paste

2 tablespoons (30 ml) coconut
aminos

2 dates, pitted

½–¾ cup (120–180 ml) water

1. Make the egg roll: Heat the coconut and sesame oils in a large skillet over medium heat. Add the cabbage, onion, and carrot and cook, stirring often, for 15–30 minutes (depending on how big your pan is), or until tender.

2. Add the ginger, garlic, and coconut aminos and cook for 5 more minutes.

3. Add the ground pork and cook, stirring regularly and breaking it up with a spatula to evenly distribute, for 10–15 minutes, or until cooked through.

4. Make the sweet and sour sauce: Heat the oil in a medium saucepan over medium heat. Add the onion and cook for about 5 minutes, or until tender. Add the garlic, salt, pepper, pineapple, tomato paste, coconut aminos, dates, and water (start with ½ cup [120 ml] and add more if needed to thin).

5. Cook for 10 minutes. Remove from the heat and blend with an immersion blender. Alternatively, you can blend it in a blender or food processor. Add more water, if needed, until the desired consistency is reached. Cook over medium heat for another 5 minutes.

6. Serve the egg roll with the sweet and sour sauce.

7. Store leftovers, covered, in the refrigerator for up to a week.

chicken alfredo–stuffed potatoes

YIELD 6-8 SERVINGS

PREP TIME 5 MINUTES

COOK TIME 50 MINUTES

EGG FREE, low LOW FODMAP,
NUT FREE IF COCONUT MILK IS USED

(IF YOU DON'T NEED LOW FODMAP,
YOU MAY USE GHEE INSTEAD OF GARLIC-
INFUSED OLIVE OIL AND ADD 1 TEA-
SPOON GARLIC POWDER TO SAUCE.)

6 medium sweet potatoes

ALFREDO SAUCE

2 tablespoons (30 ml) garlic-infused olive oil

2 tablespoons (30 g) ghee

1 heaping tablespoon (10 g) arrowroot powder

2½ cups (600 ml) almond milk

½ teaspoon salt

¼ teaspoon ground black pepper

2 tablespoons (6 g) chopped fresh chives

CHICKEN

1 tablespoon (15 ml) garlic-infused olive oil

1½-2 pounds (680-907 g) boneless skinless chicken, cut into 1-inch (3 cm) pieces

1 teaspoon salt

BROCCOLI

2 tablespoons (30 g) ghee

One 10-ounce (283 g) bag frozen broccoli

¼ teaspoon salt

This creamy chicken Alfredo and perfectly cooked broccoli are served on a baked sweet potato. The potatoes can be made ahead, making it a great weeknight meal. You could also serve chicken Alfredo over baked white potatoes instead of sweet potatoes if you prefer.

1. Preheat the oven to 400°F (200°C or gas mark 6). Line a baking sheet with parchment paper.

2. Wash and dry the sweet potatoes and place them on the prepared baking sheet. Bake for 40–50 minutes, or until fork tender.

3. While the potatoes cook, make the sauce: Heat the olive oil and ghee in a large saucepan over medium heat. Whisk in the arrowroot powder until fully combined. Add the almond milk and whisk for about 4 minutes, or until the mixture is smooth and thick. Add the salt, pepper, and chives. Leave in the pan until needed or pour into a bowl if you need the pan for the chicken.

4. Make the chicken: Heat the olive oil in a large skillet over medium heat. Add the chicken and salt and cook for 5–7 minutes, or until the chicken is cooked through. Add the chicken to the sauce.

5. Make the broccoli: Heat the ghee in a large skillet over medium heat, add the broccoli and salt, and cook, breaking the big pieces up with a spatula, for 5–7 minutes. Add to the chicken mixture and stir.

6. Remove the potatoes from the oven and cut them in half. Spoon the chicken Alfredo over the potatoes. Serve warm.

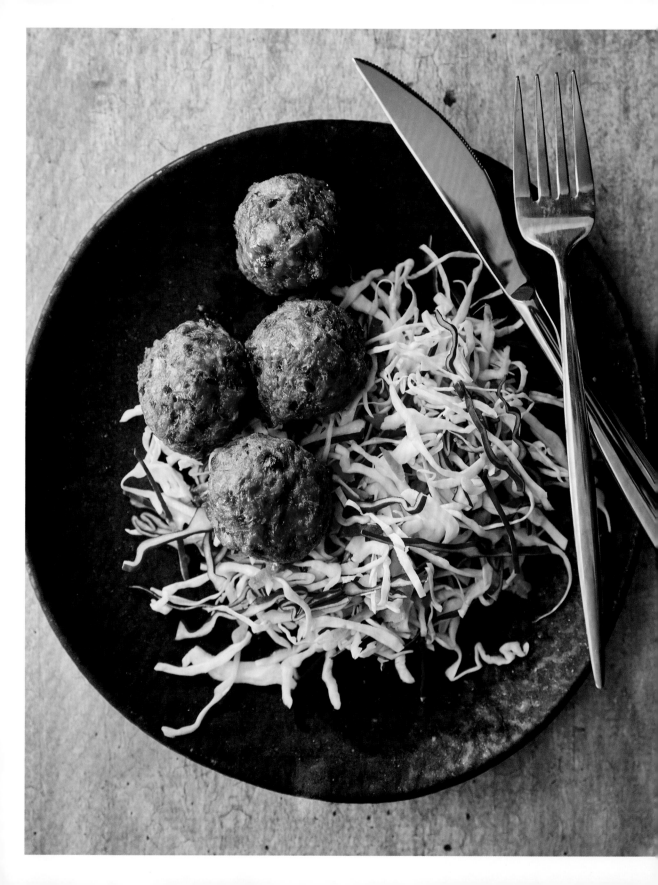

egg roll meatballs

YIELD 4 SERVINGS

PREP TIME 15 MINUTES

COOK TIME 25 MINUTES

EGG FREE, NUT FREE

All the flavors of an egg roll, packed into bite-size meatballs! Adding veggies to the meat helps bulk up the mixture and gives them great texture. The ginger, sesame oil, and coconut aminos give them an Asian-inspired taste that will satisfy any take-out craving.

One 14-ounce (392 g) bag coleslaw mix, divided

½ cup (64 g) shredded carrot

1-inch (3 cm) piece fresh ginger, peeled and grated

½ cup (64 g) diced onion

1 teaspoon salt

3 tablespoons (45 ml) coconut aminos

1 tablespoon (15 ml) toasted sesame oil

1 teaspoon garlic powder

1 pound (454 g) ground turkey or pork

1. Preheat the oven to 400°F (200°C or gas mark 6). Line a baking sheet with parchment paper.

2. Place 3 cups (180 g) of the coleslaw mix, carrot, ginger, and onion in a food processor and blend for less than 1 minute, or until the vegetables are very small and equal in size.

3. Transfer the veggie mixture to a large skillet over medium heat. Add the salt, coconut aminos, sesame oil, and garlic powder. Cook for 5 minutes, or until the vegetables are tender.

4. Transfer the veggie mixture to a large bowl. Add the ground turkey and mix well.

5. Roll into twenty-four 1-inch (3 cm) balls, arrange on the prepared baking sheet, and bake for 20 minutes.

6. Serve with the remaining coleslaw mix, if desired.

7. Store leftovers, covered, in the refrigerator for up to a week.

asian chicken thighs

YIELD 6-8 SERVINGS

PREP TIME 10 MINUTES

COOK TIME 45 MINUTES

EGG FREE, **low** LOW FODMAP,
NUT FREE

(IF YOU DON'T NEED LOW FODMAP,
YOU MAY USE 1 TEASPOON GARLIC
POWDER IN PLACE OF THE
GARLIC-INFUSED OLIVE OIL.)

6-8 bone-in skin-on chicken thighs
(about 3½ pounds [1.6 kg])

¼ cup (60 ml) coconut aminos

1 tablespoon (15 ml) toasted
sesame oil

1 tablespoon (15 ml) garlic-infused
olive oil

1 tablespoon (15 g) peeled and grated
fresh ginger

½ teaspoon red pepper flakes

1¼ teaspoons (7.5 g) salt

*These tender, juicy chicken thighs are coated in a savory sauce.
They come together quickly and make a great weeknight meal.
It's simple, but so satisfying.*

1. Preheat the oven to 400°F (200°C or gas mark 6). Place the
   chicken thighs in a 13 by 9-inch (33 by 23 cm) pan.

2. Combine the coconut aminos, sesame oil, olive oil, ginger,
   and red pepper flakes in a small bowl. Stir and pour over the
   chicken. Sprinkle the salt evenly on top of the chicken thighs.

3. Bake for 45 minutes, or until the chicken reaches 165°F (74°C)
   on a meat thermometer.

4. Serve with the sauce scooped over the chicken.

5. Store leftovers, covered, in the refrigerator for up to 6 days.

ham and pineapple chicken salad

YIELD 6-8 SERVINGS

PREP TIME 10 MINUTES

COOK TIME N/A

low LOW FODMAP, NUT FREE

(IF YOU DON'T NEED LOW FODMAP, YOU MAY USE ½ TEASPOON ONION POWDER AND ½ TEASPOON GARLIC POWDER IN PLACE OF THE CHIVES AND GARLIC-INFUSED OLIVE OIL.)

8 ounces (227 g) sugar-free ham, diced

1 pound (454 g) cooked chicken, chopped

¾ cup (180 ml) mayonnaise, homemade (page 32) or paleo store-bought

1 tablespoon (15 ml) garlic-infused olive oil

½ cup (91 g) drained canned pineapple tidbits (in juice, not syrup)

¼ teaspoon ground black pepper

2 tablespoons (6 g) chopped fresh chives

Sweet pineapple, salty ham, and tender chicken combine to make a cool meal. It's a refreshing dish that is simple and so satisfying!

1. Place the ham and chicken in a large bowl. Add the mayonnaise, olive oil, pineapple, pepper, and chives. Mix well, making sure the meat is well coated. Chill in the fridge for at least an hour and serve cold. This is great over Bibb lettuce or other greens.

2. Store leftovers, covered, in the refrigerator for up to 6 days.

Recipes

mains: beef

I love cooking with beef because it's so versatile. This chapter is heavy on the ground beef recipes because they are always quick and tasty. I think beef recipes were a staple for many people growing up. I hope to bring back those good memories through the recipes in this chapter. From meatloaf to lasagna and casseroles, all are made grain free and sugar free, but do not lack for flavor.

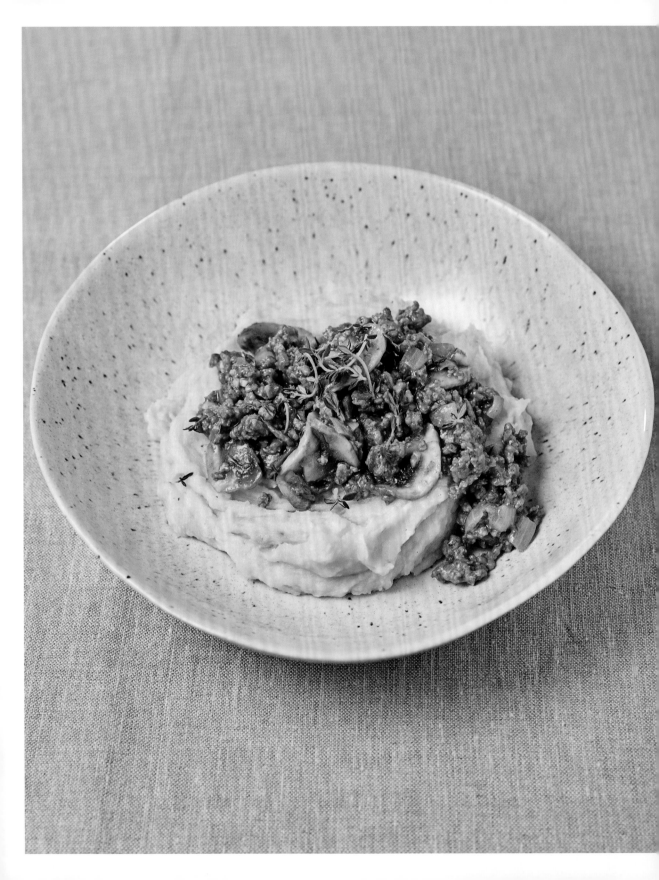

hamburger stroganoff

YIELD 6-8 SERVINGS

PREP TIME 10 MINUTES

COOK TIME 18 MINUTES

EGG FREE, NUT FREE

This stroganoff features a rich, silky sauce filled with mushrooms and ground beef. This is a no-fuss meal that is sure to be loved. It's great served over zucchini noodles or mashed potatoes!

2 tablespoons (30 ml) avocado oil

½ large onion, diced (1½ cups [192 g])

4 cloves garlic, minced

2 pounds (907 g) ground beef

2 teaspoons (12 g) salt

1 pound (454 g) mushrooms, sliced

¼ cup (60 ml) coconut aminos

1 cup (240 ml) full-fat coconut milk

2 tablespoons (20 g) arrowroot powder/starch

1 teaspoon dried thyme

1 teaspoon mild paprika

½ teaspoon ground black pepper

1. Heat the avocado oil in a large skillet over medium heat. Add the onion and garlic and cook for 5 minutes.

2. Add the beef and salt and cook, stirring regularly, for 5 minutes. Add the mushrooms and coconut aminos and cook for 5 minutes, or until the mushrooms start to soften.

3. Combine the coconut milk and arrowroot powder in a small bowl and add to the skillet. Cook for about 3 minutes, or until thick.

4. Add the thyme, paprika, and pepper and stir well. Serve immediately.

5. Store leftovers, covered, in the refrigerator for up to 6 days.

pizza meatballs

YIELD 6-8 SERVINGS

PREP TIME 20 MINUTES

COOK TIME 28 MINUTES

EGG FREE, NUT FREE

Here's everyone's favorite food turned into a meatball! These are loaded with flavor and make a great family-friendly dinner. Serve over zucchini noodles or dip them in marinara sauce.

1 pound (454 g) ground beef

1 pound (454 g) ground sugar-free Italian sausage

1 tablespoon (15 ml) avocado oil

½ cup (35 g) finely diced mushrooms

⅓ cup (43 g) diced onion

½ green pepper, diced

½ teaspoon garlic powder

½ teaspoon salt

2 ounces (57 g) pepperoni, finely diced

1 tablespoon (6 g) dried oregano

⅓ cup (80 g) marinara sauce

2 tablespoons (23 g) diced black olives (optional)

1. Preheat the oven to 375°F (190°C or gas mark 5). Line a baking sheet with parchment paper.

2. Place the beef and Italian sausage in a large bowl.

3. Heat the avocado oil in a large skillet over medium heat. Add the mushrooms, onion, green pepper, garlic powder, and salt. Cook for 5–8 minutes, or until the vegetables start to become tender. Add the vegetables to the bowl with the meat mixture.

4. Add the pepperoni, oregano, marinara sauce, and black olives, if using, to the bowl. Mix well until everything is combined.

5. Scoop a heaping tablespoon (15 g) of the mixture and roll into a ball. Place on the prepared baking sheet. Repeat until all the meatballs are rolled; it should make about 36.

6. Bake for 20 minutes. Remove from the oven and serve warm.

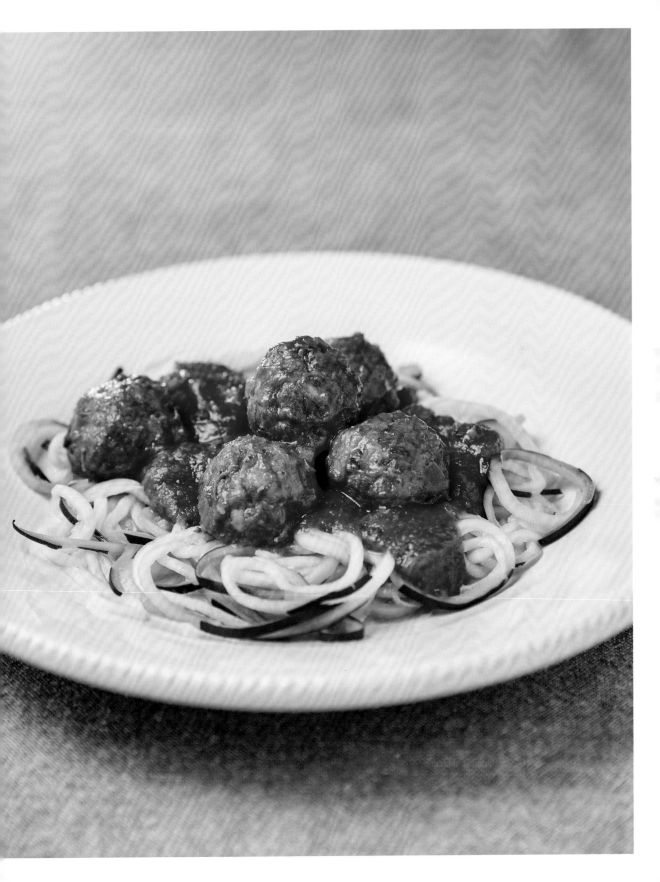

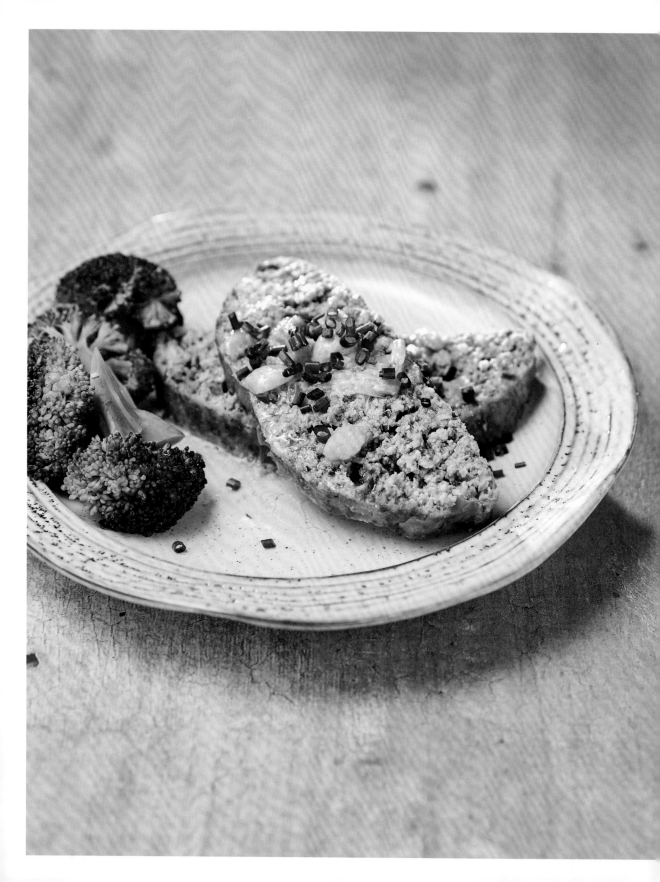

garlic lover's meatloaf

YIELD 8-10 SERVINGS

PREP TIME 20 MINUTES

COOK TIME 55 MINUTES

This is a grain-free, dairy-free take on Ina Garten's popular meat-loaf. It is moist, flavorful, and topped with an amazing garlic sauce.

MEATLOAF

2 tablespoons (30 ml) avocado oil

2 cups (256 g) chopped onion (1 large onion)

1½ cups (152 g) small-diced celery (4-6 stalks celery)

1 tablespoon (18 g) salt, divided

1 pound (454 g) ground beef

1 pound (454 g) ground turkey

1 pound (454 g) ground pork

1 tablespoon (10 g) chopped fresh parsley

1 tablespoon (6 g) chopped fresh thyme

3 large eggs

1 tablespoon (8 g) freshly ground black pepper

1 cup (112 g) almond flour

SAUCE

¾ cup (180 ml) olive oil

10-15 cloves garlic, peeled

2 cups (473 ml) chicken stock

3 tablespoons (45 ml) ghee

¼ teaspoon freshly ground black pepper

1. Preheat the oven to 350°F (180°C or gas mark 4). Line a baking sheet with parchment paper.

2. Make the meatloaf: Heat the oil in a large saucepan over medium heat. Add the onion, celery, and 1 teaspoon of the salt and cook for about 5 minutes, or until the vegetables are tender. Turn off the heat and let the mixture cool while you make the meat mixture.

3. Combine the ground beef, turkey, pork, parsley, thyme, eggs, remaining 2 teaspoons (12 g) salt, pepper, and almond flour in a large bowl. Mix well and add the onion mixture. Mix until everything is well combined.

4. Use your hands to form the meat mixture into a 14 by 5-inch (36 by 13 cm) loaf on the prepared baking sheet. Bake for 45–55 minutes, or until the temperature reaches 155°F (68°C) on a meat thermometer.

5. While the meatloaf is cooking, make the sauce: Combine the olive oil and garlic cloves in a 2-quart (2 L) saucepan. Bring the oil to a boil over high heat and then decrease the heat to low. Simmer for 10–15 minutes, or until the garlic is light golden brown. Strain out the oil and save it for another use.

6. Add the chicken stock and ghee to the same saucepan (with the garlic still in it). Bring the mixture to a boil over high heat. Lower the heat and simmer for 35–40 minutes. The sauce should be slightly thickened. Smash the garlic cloves with a fork. Add the pepper and turn off the heat.

7. Slice the meatloaf and spoon the warm sauce over it to serve.

greek meatballs

YIELD 6 SERVINGS

PREP TIME 10 MINUTES

COOK TIME 20 MINUTES

low LOW FODMAP, NUT FREE, EGG FREE

(IF YOU DON'T NEED LOW FODMAP, YOU MAY USE 1 TEASPOON ONION POWDER AND 1 TEASPOON GARLIC POWDER IN PLACE OF THE GARLIC-INFUSED OLIVE OIL AND CHIVES IN THE SAUCE.)

These meatballs are packed with spices and deliver all the flavor. The homemade tzatziki sauce really takes them over the top.

MEATBALLS

1 pound (454 g) ground beef

1 pound (454 g) ground lamb (or substitute more beef)

2 teaspoons (12 g) salt

1 teaspoon ground cumin

1 tablespoon (3 g) dried thyme

1 tablespoon (6 g) dried oregano

1 teaspoon dried rosemary

1 teaspoon ground black pepper

2 tablespoons (30 ml) garlic-infused olive oil

2 tablespoons (6 g) chopped fresh chives

TZATZIKI SAUCE

One 13.5-ounce (378 ml) can full-fat coconut milk

1 medium cucumber

2 tablespoons (30 ml) lemon juice

3 tablespoons (2 g) chopped fresh dill

½ teaspoon salt

2 teaspoons (10 ml) garlic-infused olive oil

2 tablespoons (6 g) chopped fresh chives

1. Preheat the oven to 375°F (190°C or gas mark 5). Line a baking sheet with parchment paper.

2. Make the meatballs: Combine the beef, lamb, salt, cumin, thyme, oregano, rosemary, pepper, olive oil, and chives in a large bowl. Mix well, until the spices are well distributed.

3. Form into heaping tablespoon (15 g) balls, roll between your palms, and place on the prepared baking sheet. You should get about 30 meatballs.

4. Bake for 20 minutes, or until cooked through.

5. While the meatballs are baking, make the sauce: Pour the coconut milk into a medium-size bowl. Peel and grate the cucumber and add it to the coconut milk. Add the lemon juice, dill, salt, olive oil, and chives. Whisk until smooth.

6. Serve the meatballs with the tzatziki sauce.

7. Store the meatballs and sauce, covered in separate containers, in the refrigerator for up to a week.

bolognese

YIELD 8-10 SERVINGS

PREP TIME 15 MINUTES

COOK TIME 4½ HOURS

low LOW FODMAP, NUT FREE
IF COCONUT MILK IS USED

5 strips nitrate-free bacon, cut into
½-inch (1 cm) pieces

1 tablespoon (15 ml) garlic-infused
olive oil (optional)

1 tablespoon (15 g) ghee

1 cup (96 g) chopped green onion

1 cup (128 g) diced carrots
(about 2 medium carrots)

½ cup (51 g) diced celery (2 stalks
celery)

2 pounds (907 g) ground beef

1 teaspoon salt

One 28-ounce (794 g) can crushed
tomatoes

½ cup (120 ml) coconut aminos

1 teaspoon dried oregano

½ cup (120 ml) almond milk

*This meat sauce develops great rich flavor as it slow cooks.
It's delicious served over zucchini noodles or spaghetti squash.*

1. Place the bacon in a large stockpot and cook over medium heat
   for 5–7 minutes. Add the olive oil, if needed to prevent sticking.

2. Add the ghee, green onion, carrots, and celery and cook for
   5 minutes.

3. Add the beef and salt and cook, breaking up the beef into
   small chunks, for 5–7 minutes.

4. Add the crushed tomatoes, coconut aminos, and oregano.
   Turn the heat to low, cover, and cook, stirring every 20 minutes,
   for 3–4 hours.

5. Stir in the almond milk right before serving.

6. Store leftovers, covered, in the refrigerator for up to 6 days.

lasagna

YIELD 6 SERVINGS

PREP TIME 25 MINUTES

COOK TIME 55 MINUTES

EGG FREE, **low** LOW FODMAP IF
A SENSITIVE MARINARA IS USED

(IF YOU DON'T NEED LOW FODMAP, YOU
MAY USE 1 TEASPOON GARLIC POWDER
IN PLACE OF THE OIL IN THE SAUCE.)

POTATOES

1½ pounds (680 g) sweet potatoes,
sliced ⅛ inch (3 mm) thick

1 tablespoon (15 ml) avocado oil

PASTA SAUCE

1 tablespoon (15 ml) garlic-infused
olive oil

1 pound (454 g) ground beef

1 teaspoon salt

One 24-ounce (680 g) jar sugar-free
marinara sauce

1 tablespoon (8 g) Italian seasoning

TOPPING

1 cup (112 g) almond flour

¼ teaspoon salt

1 teaspoon Italian seasoning

2 tablespoons (30 ml) melted ghee

*Sweet potatoes are used for the noodles in this hearty lasagna.
The topping tastes just like Parmesan cheese. This meal is so
satisfying and delicious.*

1. Preheat the oven to 400°F (200°C or gas mark 6). Line a baking
   sheet with parchment paper. Line a 9 by 9-inch (23 by 23 cm)
   pan with parchment paper or grease well with coconut oil.

2. Make the potatoes: Place the sweet potatoes on the prepared
   baking sheet, drizzle with the oil, and toss to coat. Spread as
   evenly as possible, but it's okay if there is some overlapping.
   Bake for 15 minutes. Decrease the oven temperature to 350°F
   (180°C or gas mark 4).

3. While potatoes are baking, make the sauce: Heat the olive oil
   in a large skillet over medium heat. Add the ground beef and
   salt and cook, breaking up the meat with a wooden spoon, for
   5 minutes.

4. Add the marinara and Italian seasoning and cook for 5–7 minutes. It should make 4 cups (960 ml) of sauce. Turn off the heat
   and set aside in the pan.

5. Make the topping: Add the almond flour, salt, Italian seasoning, and ghee to a small bowl and stir to combine. The mixture
   should be crumbly.

6. Assemble the lasagna: Place 1 cup (240 ml) pasta sauce in
   the bottom of the prepared pan, spreading evenly. Top with
   one-third of the sweet potato slices. Top with 1 cup (240 ml)
   sauce, one-third sweet potato slices, 1 cup (240 ml) sauce,
   the final one-third sweet potato slices, and the final 1 cup
   (240 ml) sauce.

7. Top with the almond flour crumble and bake for 40 minutes, or until golden brown.

8. Remove from the oven, let rest for 5 minutes, then slice and serve.

9. Store leftovers, covered, in the refrigerator for up to 6 days.

Remaking a Classic

Remaking the classic lasagna to be grain-free and cheese-free seemed like a challenge, and I was up for it. This one does not disappoint in any way. My mom made homemade lasagna a couple times of year and it was always amazing. It's a dish that does take a little extra work, but it is worth it. This version is the same. Making the sweet potatoes as the noodles takes a little time, but the payoff is great. Don't skip the topping! Since no cheese is involved, the almond-flour mixture adds great texture and a Parmesan cheese taste. This meal is satisfying and delicious, and it will become a weekend favorite!

Here is a make-ahead tip: The sweet potatoes can be prepped ahead of time in one of two ways. They can be sliced and stored, covered, in the fridge raw. They can also be sliced and cooked, then stored in the fridge so they are ready to be layered. This cuts down on the prep time on the day the lasagna is made.

spaghetti pie

YIELD 6-8 SERVINGS

PREP TIME 20 MINUTES

COOK TIME 52 MINUTES

NUT FREE, **low** LOW FODMAP
IF HOMEMADE SAUSAGE AND A
LOW-FODMAP MARINARA SUCH
AS RAO'S SENSITIVE ARE USED

1 pound (454 g) Italian sausage

1 recipe Spaghetti Squash (page 37)

One 24-ounce (680 g) jar marinara
sauce

2 large eggs

Spaghetti pie is a meal my mom used to make when I was a child. It was a "crust" of spaghetti, Parmesan, and egg filled with meat and sauce and all baked together. I loved how it had the flavors of spaghetti, but it held together and had better texture than plain spaghetti. This is a grain-free version that is just as satisfying. My mom would use ground beef, but using Italian sausage makes this so scrumptious.

1. Preheat the oven to 350°F (180°C or gas mark 4). Line a 13 by 9-inch (33 by 23 cm) pan with parchment paper or grease well with coconut oil.

2. Cook the sausage in a large skillet over medium heat for 5–7 minutes, or until it is fully cooked through.

3. Place the shredded squash in a large bowl and add the cooked sausage, marinara, and eggs. Stir well with a wooden spoon, until the squash is fully coated in sauce.

4. Pour the mixture into the prepared pan and bake for 45 minutes, or until golden brown.

5. Remove from the oven and serve immediately.

6. Store leftovers, covered, in the refrigerator for up to a week.

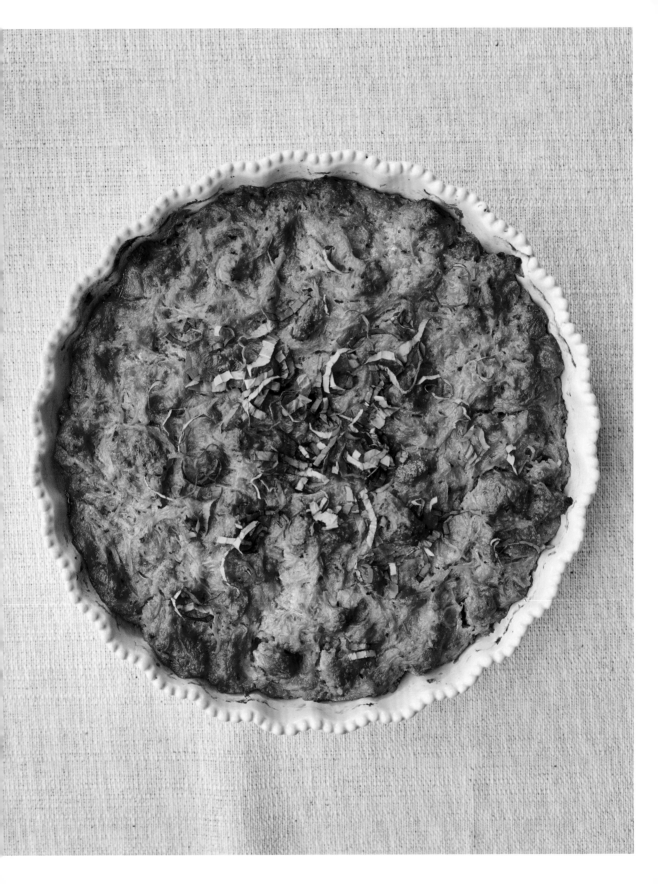

mexican skillet

YIELD 4 SERVINGS

PREP TIME 15 MINUTES

COOK TIME 25 MINUTES

EGG FREE, NUT FREE

1 tablespoon (15 ml) avocado oil

½ large onion, diced

1 bell pepper, cored and chopped

1 pound (454 g) ground beef

½ teaspoon salt

½ teaspoon ground black pepper

1 tablespoon (6 g) chili powder

1 teaspoon ground cumin

1 teaspoon paprika

1 teaspoon dried oregano

One 4-ounce (113 g) can diced green chiles

One 14.5-ounce (411 g) can fire-roasted diced tomatoes

½ cup (120 ml) water

1 pound (454 g) sweet potatoes, chopped into ½-inch (1 cm) pieces

This is a hearty one-pan meal loaded with spice. The perfectly cooked sweet potatoes balance out the savory seasonings.

1. Heat the avocado oil in a large skillet over medium heat. Add the onion and bell pepper and cook for 5 minutes. Add the beef and salt and cook, breaking up the beef with a wooden spoon, for 3 minutes.

2. Add the black pepper, chili powder, cumin, paprika, oregano, green chiles, tomatoes, water, and sweet potatoes. Stir well, cover, and cook over medium heat for 15 minutes, or until the potatoes are tender.

3. Remove from the heat and serve immediately.

4. Store leftovers, covered, in the refrigerator for up to 6 days.

chili dog casserole

YIELD 8–10 SERVINGS

PREP TIME 20 MINUTES

COOK TIME 1 HOUR 15 MINUTES

EGG FREE, NUT FREE

This is a fun and pleasing meal the whole family will love. Chili and hot dogs make the first layer, topped with creamy mashed potatoes.

BEEF LAYER

1 pound (454 g) ground beef

1 teaspoon salt

1 large onion, diced

4 cloves garlic, minced

One 25-ounce (709 g) can crushed tomatoes

One 14.5-ounce (411 g) can diced tomatoes

¼ cup (24 g) chili powder

6 nitrate-free hot dogs (such as Teton Water Ranch or Applegate), cut into ½-inch (1 cm) slices

MASHED POTATO TOPPING

3 pounds (1.4 kg) Yukon gold potatoes

½ teaspoon salt

1 cup (240 ml) chicken broth

½ teaspoon garlic powder

¼ teaspoon ground black pepper

1. Make the beef mixture: Place the beef and salt in a large skillet and cook over medium heat, breaking it apart as it cooks, for 5 minutes.

2. Add the onion and garlic and cook for 5 minutes.

3. Add the tomatoes, chili powder, and hot dogs and cook over low heat for 20–30 minutes.

4. While the beef mixture cooks, make the mashed potatoes: Wash and cut the potatoes into fourths. Place the potatoes in a 2-quart (2 L) pot, cover with cold water, and add the salt. Turn the heat to medium-high and stir occasionally until the water boils. This should take 8–10 minutes.

5. Cover, turn the heat to low, and cook for 10–15 minutes, or until a fork can easily pierce a potato.

6. Turn off the heat, drain the potatoes, and return them to the hot pot. Add the chicken broth, garlic powder, and pepper and mash with a potato masher until smooth.

7. Preheat the oven to 375°F (190°C or gas mark 5). Line a 13 by 9-inch (33 by 23 cm) pan with parchment paper or grease well with coconut oil.

8. Place the chili dog mixture in the bottom of the prepared pan and top evenly with the mashed potatoes, spreading them to the edges. Bake for 30 minutes.

9. Remove from the oven and serve immediately.

10. Store leftovers, covered, in the refrigerator for up to 6 days.

barbecue shredded beef

YIELD 6 SERVINGS

PREP TIME 10 MINUTES

COOK TIME 3½ HOURS

EGG FREE, NUT FREE

Tender beef paired with savory barbecue sauce makes this meal uncomplicated and so darn good. It's great served with baked sweet or white potatoes.

1 tablespoon (15 ml) avocado oil

1 large onion, chopped

1½ pounds (680 g) beef roast, cut into 2-inch (5 cm) chunks

1 teaspoon salt

1 cup (240 ml) barbecue sauce, homemade (page 35) or paleo store-bought

¼ cup (60 ml) coconut aminos

1. Heat the avocado oil in a small Dutch oven over medium heat. Add the onion and cook for 5 minutes. Add the beef, salt, barbecue sauce, and coconut aminos and stir to combine.

2. Decrease the heat to low, cover, and cook, stirring every 30 minutes, for 2½ hours. Uncover and cook, stirring regularly and breaking up large chunks of meat, for 1 more hour. Serve.

3. Store leftovers, covered, in the refrigerator for up to 6 days.

korean shredded beef

YIELD 4 SERVINGS

PREP TIME 10 MINUTES

COOK TIME 55 MINUTES

EGG FREE, NUT FREE

1-1¼ pounds (454–568 g) flank steak, cut against the grain into fourths

¼ cup (60 ml) coconut aminos

2 teaspoons (10 ml) toasted sesame oil

½ large onion, chopped

3 cloves garlic, minced

1 teaspoon ground ginger

½ teaspoon red pepper flakes

¼ teaspoon salt

This beef has Asian flair from the ginger, sesame oil, and coconut aminos. It's bursting with flavor and so tender and delicious. Serve over a bowl of greens or in grain-free tortillas.

1. Place the beef in the electric pressure cooker. Add the coconut aminos, sesame oil, onion, garlic, ginger, red pepper flakes, and salt. Stir to combine.

2. Place the lid on, close the valve, and cook on High for 40 minutes. Let naturally release for 15 minutes; this helps the meat stay juicy.

3. Press Cancel, release the valve, and open the lid. Press Sauté and cook, stirring to help shred the meat, for 8–10 minutes. The juices should reduce. Serve immediately.

4. Store leftovers, covered, in the refrigerator for up to a week.

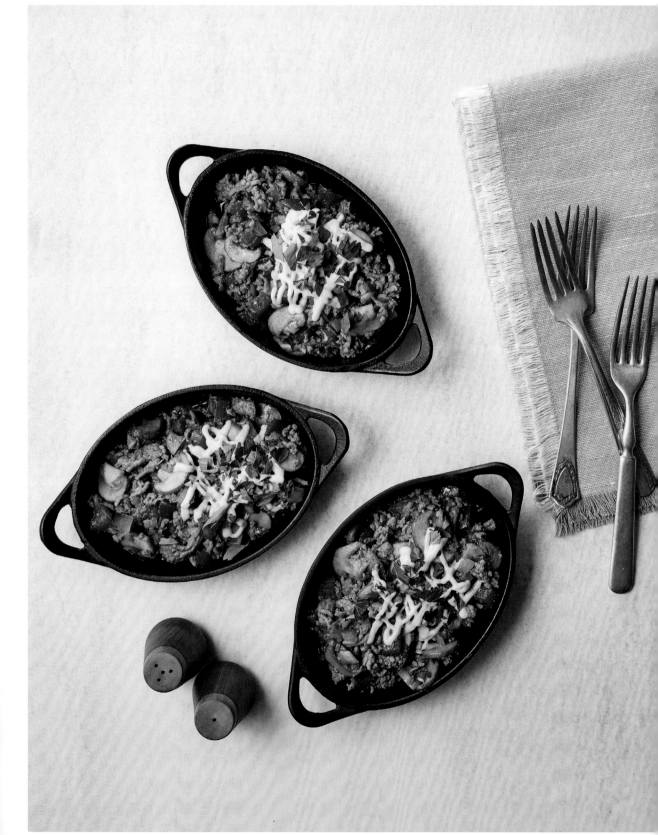

philly cheesesteak skillet

YIELD 6-8 SERVINGS

PREP TIME 15 MINUTES

COOK TIME 30 MINUTES

EGG FREE, NUT FREE

Using ground beef is a shortcut that makes this dish come together quickly. The mayo topping is in place of the traditional cheese and adds great creaminess.

SKILLET

2 tablespoons (30 ml) avocado oil

1 large onion, chopped

1½ pounds (680 g) mushrooms, sliced

3 green peppers, cored and chopped

2 teaspoons (12 g) salt, divided

2 pounds (907 g) ground beef

2 tablespoons (30 ml) coconut aminos

1 teaspoon garlic powder

2 tablespoons (20 g) arrowroot powder/starch

TOPPING

1 cup (240 ml) mayonnaise, homemade (page 32) or paleo store-bought

2 tablespoons (30 ml) coconut aminos

¼ teaspoon garlic powder

¼ teaspoon onion powder

1. Make the skillet: Heat the avocado oil in a large skillet over medium heat. Add the onion, mushrooms, peppers, and 1 teaspoon of the salt and cook, stirring regularly, for 10 minutes.

2. Add the ground beef, remaining 1 teaspoon salt, coconut aminos, and garlic powder. Cook for 10–15 minutes, or until the meat is fully cooked and the vegetables are tender. Sprinkle in the arrowroot powder and stir well for 3–5 minutes, or until thick.

3. Make the topping: Combine the mayonnaise, coconut aminos, garlic powder, and onion powder in a small bowl. Drizzle over the skillet when serving.

sheet pan garlic steak and potatoes

YIELD 6-8 SERVINGS

PREP TIME 15 MINUTES

COOK TIME 52 MINUTES

EGG FREE, `low` LOW FODMAP, NUT FREE

(IF YOU DON'T NEED LOW FODMAP, YOU MAY USE AVOCADO OIL ON THE STEAK WITH ½ TEASPOON GARLIC POWDER INSTEAD OF THE GARLIC-INFUSED OIL.)

2 pounds (907 g) potatoes, cut into 1-inch (3 cm) chunks

1 tablespoon (15 ml) avocado oil

2 teaspoons (12 g) salt, divided

2 pounds (907 g) steak, cut into ½ by 1 inch (1 by 3 cm) pieces

1 tablespoon (15 ml) garlic-infused olive oil

An irresistible combination of crispy potatoes and perfectly cooked bites of tender steak. My daughter is a little bit of a picky eater, but she never turns down steak or any form of potatoes. She absolutely loved this meal, and I love how easy it is. There's nothing fancy or complicated with this dish, but it's classic comfort food.

1. Preheat the oven to 425°F (220°C or gas mark 7). Line a baking sheet with parchment paper.

2. Place the potatoes on the baking sheet, drizzle with the avocado oil, add 1 teaspoon of the salt, and toss to coat. Bake for 40 minutes.

3. Remove from the oven and push the potatoes to one side of the baking sheet. Add the steak in an even layer on the other side. Drizzle with the olive oil and remaining 1 teaspoon salt. Toss to coat evenly.

4. Bake for 9–12 minutes, or until the steak is done to your liking.

5. Remove from the oven and serve immediately.

6. Store leftovers, covered, in the refrigerator for up to 6 days.

classic meatloaf

YIELD 8-10 SERVINGS

PREP TIME 15 MINUTES

COOK TIME 1 HOUR 30 MINUTES

MEATLOAF

1 tablespoon (15 ml) avocado oil

1 large onion, diced

2 pounds (907 g) grass-fed ground beef

1 cup (113 g) cooked sweet potato

1 cup (112 g) almond flour

2 tablespoons (15 g) coconut flour

1 large egg, at room temperature

1 cup (240 ml) ketchup, homemade (page 33) or paleo store-bought

3 tablespoons (45 ml) coconut aminos

2 teaspoons (12 g) salt

1 teaspoon (3 g) garlic powder

GLAZE

½ cup (120 ml) ketchup, homemade (page 33) or paleo store-bought

2 tablespoons (30 ml) coconut aminos

This is a traditional meatloaf given a healthy makeover. Sweet potato is added for bulk and nutrition, and almond flour is used in place of breadcrumbs. This is a big loaf, so it's best made when you have a little extra time. Leftovers are even better, though, making this a great meal to have on hand for the week.

1. Preheat the oven to 350°F (180°C or gas mark 4). Line a rimmed baking sheet with parchment paper.

2. Make the meatloaf: Heat the oil in a large skillet over medium heat. Add the onion and sauté for 5–7 minutes, or until softened and translucent.

3. In a large bowl, mix the beef, onion, sweet potato, almond flour, coconut flour, egg, ketchup, coconut aminos, salt, and garlic powder with your hands until just combined. Don't overmix, or the meat can become tough.

4. Form the mixture into a loaf shape on the prepared baking sheet.

5. Make the glaze: Mix the ketchup and coconut aminos in a small bowl and spoon on top of the meatloaf.

6. Bake for 60 minutes. Remove from the oven and carefully scoop the grease into a jar or bowl and discard.

7. Return the meatloaf to the oven and bake for 30 minutes longer, or until the meatloaf reaches 160°F–165°F (71°C–74°C) on a meat thermometer.

8. Remove from the oven, let rest for a few minutes, then slice and serve.

9. Store leftovers, covered, in the refrigerator for up to 6 days.

Recipes

Chapter 8

---

soups

As soon as the air gets a little chill to it, I start craving soups. They are definitely among the most comforting meals! The flavor options for soups are endless, and they are usually easy to make. Leftovers are just as good or better, and they are always a good option for serving a crowd. I tried to cover all the bases here, from spicy to creamy to kid-friendly.

taco soup

YIELD 4-6 SERVINGS

PREP TIME 10 MINUTES

COOK TIME 20 MINUTES

EGG FREE, NUT FREE

This recipe combines two beloved dishes—tacos and soup—into one meal. It's quick to make, hearty, and freezes wonderfully. This is sure to become a fall and winter staple.

1 tablespoon (15 ml) avocado oil

1 large onion, diced

1 bell pepper, cored and chopped

1 pound (454 g) ground beef

2 tablespoons (12 g) chili powder

1 tablespoon (8 g) ground cumin

1 teaspoon salt

1 teaspoon ground black pepper

1 teaspoon paprika

½ teaspoon garlic powder

½ teaspoon onion powder

1 teaspoon dried oregano

4 cups (946 ml) beef broth

One 14.5-ounce (411 g) can diced tomatoes

One 4-ounce (113 g) can diced green chiles

1. Heat the avocado oil in a large stockpot over medium heat. Add the onion, bell pepper, and ground beef and cook for 5 minutes.

2. Add the chili powder, cumin, salt, pepper, paprika, garlic powder, onion powder, oregano, broth, tomatoes, and chiles. Stir well and cook for 15 minutes, or until the veggies are tender.

3. Ladle into bowls and serve.

4. Store leftovers, covered, in the refrigerator for up to a week.

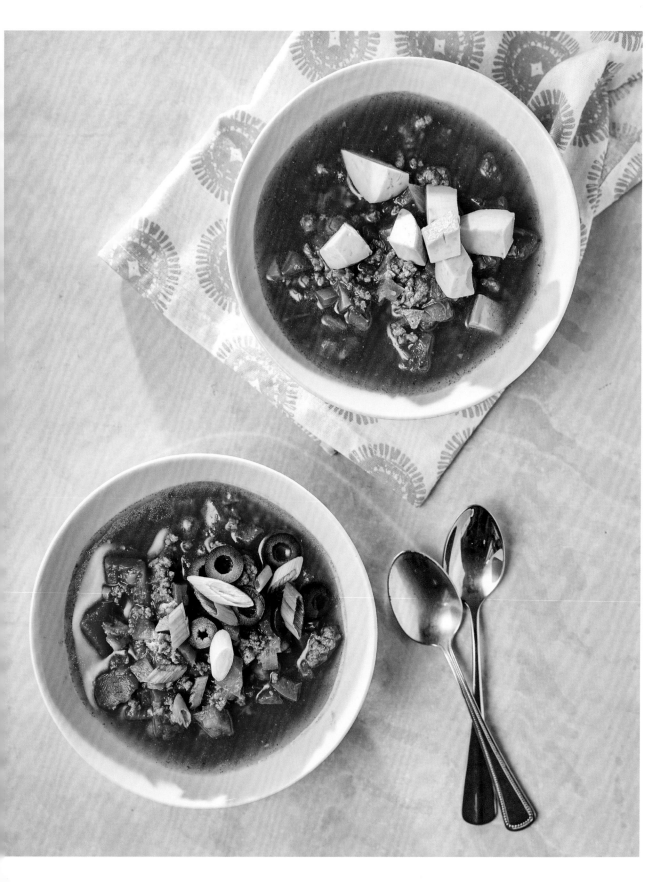

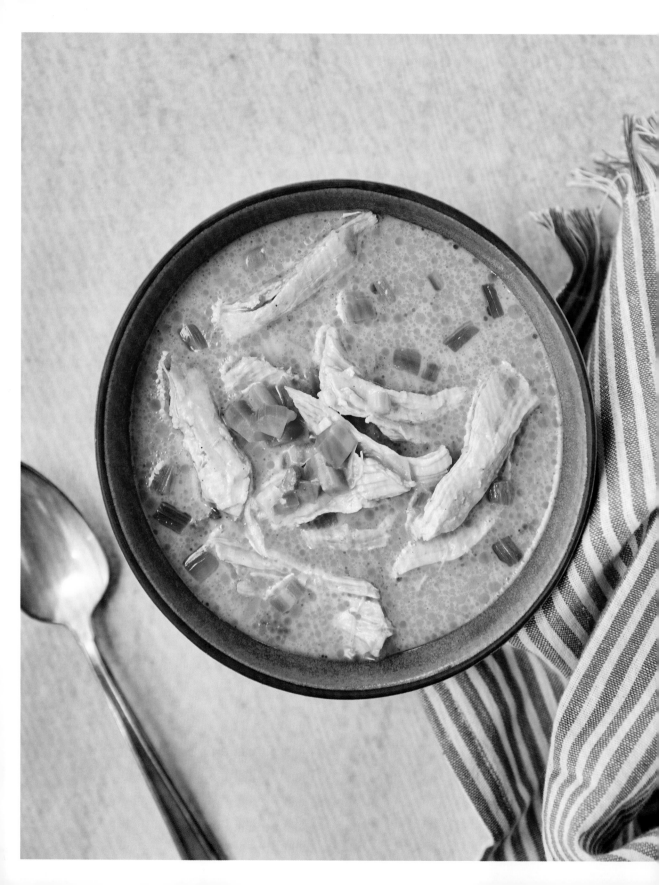

buffalo chicken soup

YIELD 4–6 SERVINGS

PREP TIME 15 MINUTES

COOK TIME 30 MINUTES

NUT FREE

Imagine all the flavors of a buffalo wing, but in soup form. This soup is spiced just right—not too hot—and the ranch dressing gives it a cool creaminess.

2 tablespoons (30 g) ghee

1 cup (120 g) diced celery

3 large carrots, chopped
(about 1½ cups [192 g])

1 large onion, diced

3 or 4 cloves garlic, minced

½ teaspoon salt

1–1½ pounds (454–680 g) boneless
skinless chicken

¼ cup (60 ml) cayenne pepper sauce,
such as Frank's RedHot

4 cups (946 ml) chicken broth

⅓ cup (80 ml) ranch dressing,
homemade (page 36) or paleo
store-bought

1. Heat the ghee in a large stockpot over medium heat. Add the celery, carrots, onion, garlic, and salt. Cook, stirring regularly, for 5 minutes.

2. Add the chicken, pepper sauce, and broth. Decrease the heat to medium-low, cover, and cook for 15 minutes, or until the chicken is fully cooked through.

3. Transfer the chicken to a cutting board and chop into bite-size pieces. Return the chicken to the broth and add the ranch dressing. Stir well. Cook over medium heat for 5–10 more minutes, or until fully warmed though.

4. Ladle into bowls and serve.

5. Store leftovers, covered, in the refrigerator for up to 6 days.

french onion soup with meatballs

YIELD 8 SERVINGS

PREP TIME 15 MINUTES

COOK TIME 1 HOUR 10 MINUTES

NUT FREE

The classic French onion soup is taken to the next level with the addition of tender meatballs. Doing so makes it a complete meal, and they pair perfectly together. The onions take a little time to cook down, but it's worth it because they become beautifully caramelized and sweet.

SOUP

¼ cup (60 g) ghee

6 sweet onions, sliced

1 teaspoon salt

3 cloves garlic, minced

1 tablespoon (6 g) chopped fresh thyme

7 cups (1.7 L) beef broth

3 tablespoons (45 ml) coconut aminos

MEATBALLS

2 pounds (907 g) ground beef

1 teaspoon salt

1 teaspoon dried thyme

1 teaspoon garlic powder

1 teaspoon onion powder

1 large egg

2 tablespoons (30 ml) coconut aminos

1. Heat the ghee in a large stock pot over medium-low heat. Add the onions and salt and cook, stirring regularly, for 50–55 minutes, or until the onions are browned and cooked down.

2. While the onions are cooking, make the meatballs: Preheat the oven to 400°F (200°C or gas mark 6). Line a baking sheet with parchment paper.

3. Combine the ground beef, salt, thyme, garlic powder, onion powder, egg, and coconut aminos in a large bowl. Mix well.

4. Scoop the mixture into heaping tablespoons (15 g) and roll into about 35 balls. Place the balls on the prepared baking sheet. Bake for 18 minutes. Remove from the oven and set aside still on the baking sheet until ready to add to the soup.

5. When the onions are done, add the garlic and thyme and cook for 5 minutes. Add the broth, coconut aminos, and meatballs and cook over medium heat for 10 minutes.

6. Ladle into bowls and serve immediately, making sure to get onions and meatballs in every bowl.

7. Store leftovers, covered, in the refrigerator for up to 6 days.

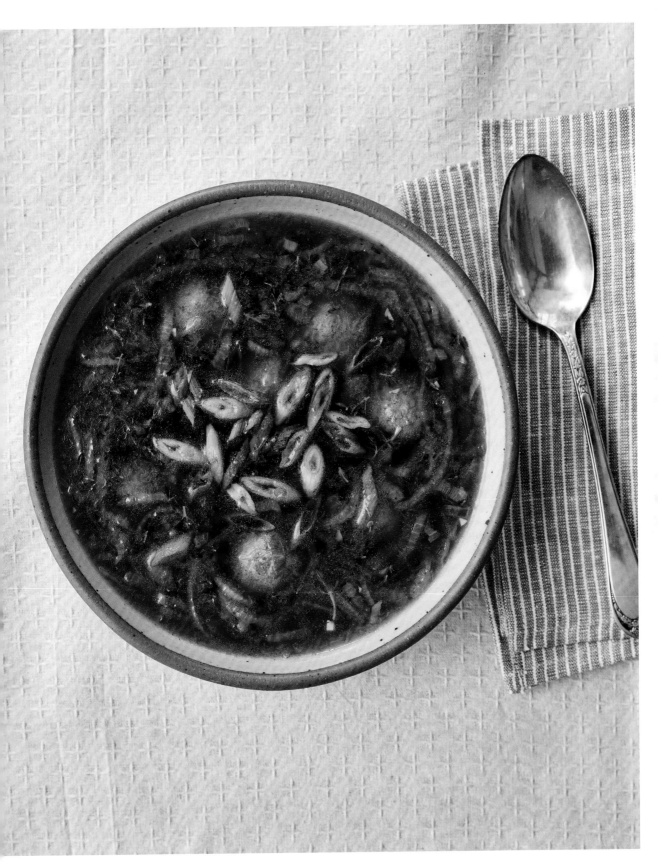

sloppy joe soup

YIELD 6–8 SERVINGS

PREP TIME 10 MINUTES

COOK TIME 30 MINUTES

low LOW FODMAP IF LOW-FODMAP KETCHUP IS USED

(IF YOU DON'T NEED LOW FODMAP, YOU MAY USE ANY PALEO KETCHUP, SWEET ONION IN PLACE OF GREEN ONION, AND 1 TEASPOON GARLIC POWDER IN PLACE OF THE GARLIC-INFUSED OLIVE OIL.)

1 tablespoon (15 ml) garlic-infused olive oil

2 bell peppers, cored and chopped

¼ cup (24 g) diced green onion

1 teaspoon salt

2 pounds (907 g) ground beef

1½ cups (355 ml) ketchup, homemade (page 33) or paleo store-bought

½ cup (120 ml) coconut aminos

3 cups (720 ml) water

1½ pounds (680 g) sweet potatoes, cut into ½-inch (1 cm) cubes

My Sloppy Joe recipe is one of the most popular recipes on my website. I took the idea of this childhood classic and turned it into a soup, and it came out wonderfully. It's savory, hearty, and irresistible.

1. Heat the olive oil in a large stockpot over medium heat. Add the peppers, green onion, and salt and cook for 5 minutes.

2. Add the ground beef, ketchup, and coconut aminos and stir to combine. Cook, breaking up the meat with a wooden spoon, for 5 minutes.

3. Add the water and sweet potatoes. Cover and cook for 15–20 minutes, or until the potatoes are tender.

4. Ladle into bowls and serve immediately.

5. Store leftovers, covered, in the refrigerator for up to a week.

hamburger soup

YIELD 6 SERVINGS

PREP TIME 15 MINUTES

COOK TIME 30 MINUTES

EGG FREE, NUT FREE

1 tablespoon (15 ml) avocado oil

1 cup (120 g) chopped celery

1 red bell pepper, cored and diced

1 large onion, diced

1 pound (454 g) ground beef

4 cups (946 ml) beef broth

1 cup (240 ml) water

1 cup (128 g) sliced carrots

1½ pounds (680 g) potatoes, cut into ½-inch (1 cm) chunks

One 14.5-ounce (411 g) can diced tomatoes

2 tablespoons (30 ml) coconut aminos

2 teaspoons (5 g) Italian seasoning

1 teaspoon garlic powder

This is a soup that comes together quickly and is sure to be a hit. It's packed with veggies and seasoning. A great simple dinner!

1. Heat the avocado oil in a large stockpot over medium heat. Add the celery, pepper, and onion and cook for 5 minutes.

2. Add the beef and cook for 3 minutes.

3. Add the broth, water, carrots, potatoes, tomatoes, coconut aminos, Italian seasoning, and garlic powder. Stir to combine.

4. Bring to a boil over high heat, decrease the heat to medium-low, cover, and cook for 15–20 minutes, or until the potatoes are tender.

5. Ladle into bowls and serve immediately.

6. Store leftovers, covered, in the refrigerator for up to a week.

chicken feel-good soup

YIELD 6-8 SERVINGS

PREP TIME 15 MINUTES

COOK TIME 25 MINUTES

EGG FREE, low LOW FODMAP, NUT FREE

(IF YOU DON'T NEED LOW FODMAP, YOU MAY USE A SMALL SWEET ONION IN PLACE OF THE GREEN ONION AND 3 CLOVES FRESH MINCED GARLIC IN PLACE OF THE GARLIC-INFUSED OLIVE OIL. USE MORE GHEE IN PLACE OF THE GARLIC-INFUSED OLIVE OIL.)

2 tablespoons (30 ml) garlic-infused olive oil

1 tablespoon (15 g) ghee

1 pound (454 g) carrots, sliced into ¼-inch (6 mm)-thick pieces (about 3 cups)

⅔ cup (64 g) chopped green onion

2-inch (5 cm) piece fresh ginger, peeled and grated

1½ teaspoons (9 g) salt

6 cups (1.4 L) water

1 teaspoon turmeric

¼ teaspoon ground black pepper

1½ pounds (680 g) boneless skinless chicken thighs

This is the soup you need to make when you feel a cold coming on—or you just need a hug in a bowl. The fresh ginger and turmeric are anti-inflammatory foods that will help you heal.

1. Heat the olive oil and ghee in a large stockpot over medium heat. Add the carrots, green onion, ginger, and salt. Cook for 3 minutes.

2. Add the water, turmeric, pepper, and chicken. Bring to a boil over high heat and cook for about 5 minutes, then decrease the heat to medium-low, cover, and cook for 15 minutes.

3. Remove the chicken and place on a cutting board. Chop into bite-size pieces and return to the soup. Cook for 5 more minutes.

4. Ladle into bowls and serve immediately.

5. Store leftovers, covered, in the refrigerator for up to 6 days.

beef stew

YIELD 6-8 SERVINGS

PREP TIME 15 MINUTES

COOK TIME 3 HOURS

EGG FREE, **low** LOW FODMAP, NUT FREE

(IF YOU DON'T NEED LOW FODMAP, YOU MAY USE A SMALL SWEET ONION IN PLACE OF THE GREEN ONION. USE AVOCADO OIL IN PLACE OF THE GARLIC-INFUSED OLIVE OIL AND ADD 1 TEASPOON GARLIC POWDER.)

2 tablespoons (30 ml) garlic-infused olive oil, divided

2 pounds (907 g) stew meat or roast cut into 1-inch (3 cm) chunks, divided

1½ teaspoons (9 g) salt, divided

⅓ cup (32 g) chopped green onion

¼ cup (60 ml) coconut aminos

One 14.5-ounce (411 g) can diced tomatoes

3 cups (720 ml) water

2 teaspoons (4 g) chopped fresh thyme

1 cup (120 g) chopped celery

2 cups (300 g) chopped carrots (about 3 carrots)

1 pound (454 g) potatoes, cut into ½-inch (1 cm) chunks

The ingredients are simple, and there is something so nicely familiar about beef stew. This one is just like you remember—hearty, thick, and full of tender beef.

1. Heat 1 tablespoon (15 ml) of the olive oil in a large stockpot or Dutch oven over medium-high heat. Add 1 pound (454 g) of the meat and ½ teaspoon (3 g) of the salt and cook for about 5 minutes, or until the meat is browned on all sides. Transfer to a plate and repeat with the remaining 1 tablespoon (15 ml) oil, remaining 1 pound (454 g) meat, and ½ teaspoon (3 g) salt.

2. Return the first batch of beef to the pan. Add the green onion, coconut aminos, tomatoes, water, thyme, and remaining ½ teaspoon (3 g) salt. Decrease the heat to low, cover, and cook, stirring every 30 minutes, for 2 hours.

3. Add the celery, carrots, and potatoes, cover, and cook for 40–50 minutes, or until all the veggies are tender.

4. Ladle into bowls and serve immediately.

5. Store leftovers, covered, in the refrigerator for up to 6 days.

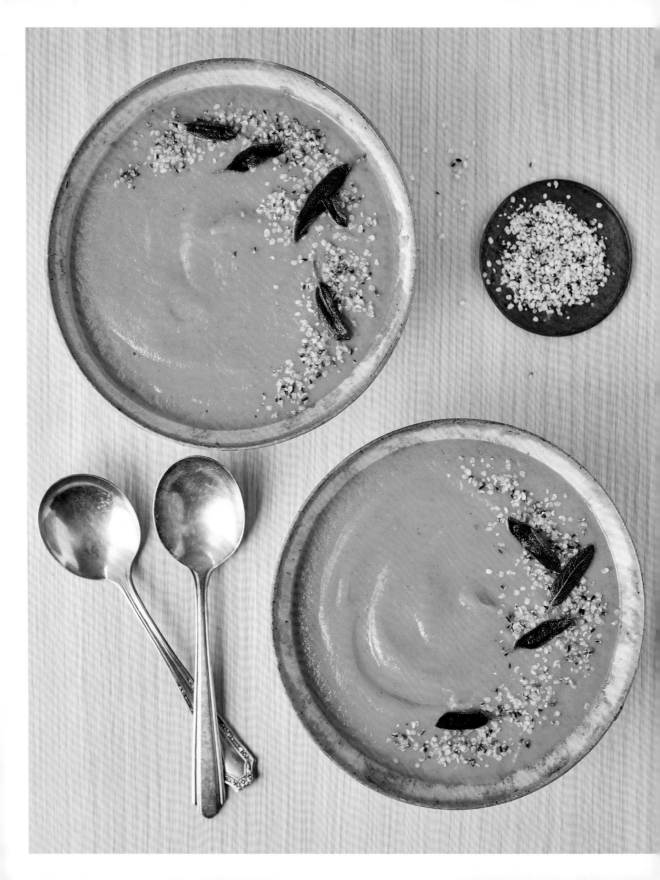

carrot ginger soup

YIELD 8–10 SERVINGS

PREP TIME 15 MINUTES

COOK TIME 30 MINUTES

EGG FREE, **low** LOW FODMAP, NUT FREE

4 pounds (1.8 kg) carrots

4-inch (10 cm) piece fresh ginger, peeled and sliced

1 teaspoon salt

7 cups (1.7 L) water

15–20 fresh sage leaves, divided

¼ cup (60 ml) avocado oil, divided

¼ cup (60 g) ghee, divided

This soup is creamy, thick, and delightful. There is a subtle kick from the ginger that is balanced by the carrots' sweetness. This is great served as a side dish to roasted chicken. Also, this is one of my daughter's favorite recipes to help me with. All those carrots to peel and cut? It's fun to have someone help!

1. Peel the carrots, cut off the ends, and cut into 1-inch (3 cm) chunks. Cut larger carrot pieces in half widthwise as well. Place the carrots in a large stockpot. Add the ginger, salt, and water.

2. Bring the mixture to a boil over high heat, which takes about 15 minutes. Decrease the heat to medium-low and cook for about 20 minutes, or until the carrots are tender.

3. Remove the pot from the heat. Place half the mixture in a high-powdered blender, add half of the sage, 2 tablespoons (30 ml) of the avocado oil, and 2 tablespoons (30 g) of the ghee. Blend until smooth and creamy. When blending a hot liquid, remove the top piece on the lid of the blender and cover with a kitchen towel. This will let the heat release safely.

4. Pour the blended soup into a bowl and repeat with the remaining half of the carrot mixture, remaining half of the sage, remaining 2 tablespoons (30 ml) avocado oil, and remaining 2 tablespoons (30 g) ghee. Blend and pour into the same bowl as the first batch. Stir.

5. Ladle into bowls and serve immediately.

6. Store leftovers, covered, in the refrigerator for up to a week.

ham and potato soup

YIELD 4-6 SERVINGS

PREP TIME 15 MINUTES

COOK TIME 30 MINUTES

NUT FREE IF COCONUT MILK
IS USED INSTEAD OF ALMOND MILK

Tender potatoes and veggies combine with chunks of ham to make this soup irresistible. Blending the potatoes partially makes it amazingly creamy.

1 tablespoon (15 ml) avocado oil

2 cups (223 g) diced celery

1¼ cups (170 g) diced carrots
(about 2 medium carrots)

1½ cups (183 g) diced onion
(about ½ large onion)

1½ pounds (680 g) potatoes,
peeled and chopped into ½-inch
(1 cm) pieces (about 4 cups [637 g])

4 cups (946 ml) unsalted chicken
broth

1 cup (240 ml) water

1 teaspoon garlic powder

1 teaspoon chopped fresh thyme

¼ teaspoon ground black pepper

1 cup (240 ml) almond milk

2½ ounces kale, chopped (5 cups
[71 g])

1 pound (454 g) chopped ham

Salt to taste

1. Heat the avocado oil in a large stockpot over medium heat. Add the celery, carrots, and onion and cook for 5–7 minutes, or until they start to get tender.

2. Add the potatoes, broth, water, garlic powder, thyme, and black pepper and bring to a boil over high heat. Decrease the heat to medium-low and cook for 15 minutes, or until the potatoes are tender.

3. Turn off the heat and add the almond milk. Blend the soup slightly with an immersion blender, making it creamy while still leaving chunks of potatoes.

4. Add the kale and ham and cook for 5 minutes, or until the kale is wilted. Taste and add salt if needed. Serve warm.

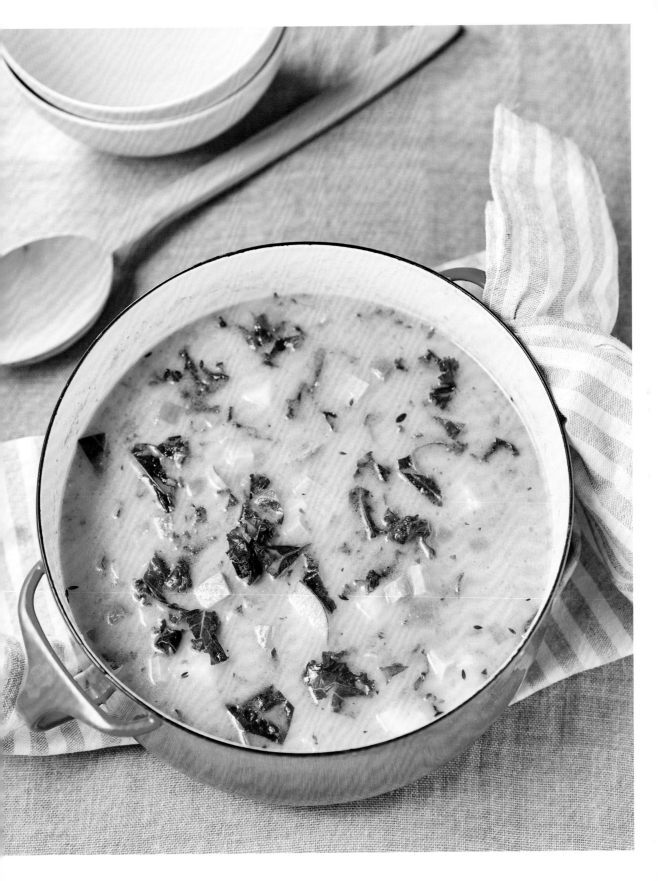

spicy chicken soup

YIELD 8 SERVINGS

PREP TIME 15 MINUTES

COOK TIME 30 MINUTES

EGG FREE, NUT FREE

1 large onion, diced

1 pound (454 g) spicy ground sausage or chorizo

1 pound (454 g) boneless skinless chicken thighs, cut into ½-inch (1 cm) pieces

Two 14.5-ounce (411 g) cans diced tomatoes

One 4-ounce (113 g) can diced green chiles

4 cups (946 ml) chicken broth

¼ teaspoon salt

1 tablespoon (8 g) ground cumin

1 tablespoon (6 g) dried oregano

1 tablespoon (7 g) paprika

½ teaspoon (1 g) ground black pepper

This soup is bursting with rich, deep flavor. It comes together quickly, making it great for a weeknight meal.

1. Place the onion and sausage in a large stockpot over medium heat and cook, breaking up the sausage with a wooden spoon, for 5 minutes.

2. Add the chicken and cook for 3 minutes.

3. Add the tomatoes, chiles, broth, salt, cumin, oregano, paprika, and pepper. Cook over medium-low heat for 20–25 minutes, or until the chicken is cooked through.

4. Ladle into bowls and serve immediately.

5. Store leftovers, covered, in the refrigerator for up to 6 days.

clam chowder

YIELD 4–6 SERVINGS

PREP TIME 15 MINUTES

COOK TIME 30 MINUTES

EGG FREE, **low** LOW FODMAP,
NUT FREE IF COCONUT MILK IS
USED INSTEAD OF ALMOND MILK

My sister was super excited when I made this dairy-free, creamy soup. It was a favorite of hers before she ate paleo, and she loves how much this one tastes like the original. The pureed potatoes give it amazing creaminess—you won't miss the dairy at all.

2 tablespoons (30 g) ghee

1 bunch green onions, chopped
(½ cup [48 g])

¾ cup (76 g) chopped celery

¼ teaspoon salt

2 pounds (907 g) potatoes,
cut into ½-inch (1 cm) chunks

2 cups (473 ml) chicken broth

1 cup (240 ml) almond milk

Three 6.5-ounce (184 g) cans
clams, including the juice

½ cup (120 ml) clam juice

1. Heat the ghee in a large stockpot over medium heat. Add the green onions, celery, and salt and cook for 5 minutes, or until the vegetables start to soften.

2. Add the potatoes and broth and cook for 20 minutes, or until the potatoes are tender. Transfer 2½–3 cups (600–720 ml) of potatoes (a little liquid is fine) to a blender, add the almond milk, and blend until smooth.

3. Return the potato mixture to the soup, add the clams and clam juice, and cook over medium heat for 5 more minutes.

4. Ladle into bowls and serve immediately.

5. Store leftovers, covered, in the refrigerator for up to 6 days.

creamy crab soup

YIELD 4 SERVINGS

PREP TIME 10 MINUTES

COOK TIME 30 MINUTES

EGG FREE, **low** LOW FODMAP IF NEW BAE (NOT OLD BAY) SEASONING IS USED, NUT FREE

(IF YOU DON'T NEED LOW FODMAP, YOU MAY USE A SMALL SWEET ONION IN PLACE OF THE GREEN ONION. USE MORE GHEE AND 1 TEASPOON GARLIC POWDER IN PLACE OF THE GARLIC-INFUSED OIL.)

1 tablespoon (15 ml) garlic-infused olive oil

1 tablespoon (15 g) ghee

1 bunch green onions, chopped (½ cup [48 g])

1 cup (142 g) diced carrot

One 14.5-ounce (411 g) can fire-roasted diced tomatoes

2 cups (473 ml) water

2 teaspoons (12 g) Primal Palate New Bae Seasoning

1 cup (240 ml) full-fat coconut milk

Two 4.25-ounce (120 g) cans white lump crab

2 tablespoons (30 ml) lemon juice

A rich, creamy soup with chunks of tender crabmeat, this is a light meal that is still filling. It comes together quickly, and the crab flavor is not overpowering.

1. Heat the olive oil and ghee in a large stockpot over medium heat. Add the green onions and carrot and cook for 3–4 minutes.

2. Add the tomatoes, water, and seasoning. Bring to a boil over high heat, decrease the heat to medium-low, and cook for 10–15 minutes.

3. Add the coconut milk and turn off the heat. Blend with an immersion blender until smooth.

4. Add the crab and lemon juice and cook over medium heat for 5 minutes.

5. Ladle into bowls and serve immediately.

6. Store leftovers, covered, in the refrigerator for up to 6 days.

broccoli cheese soup

YIELD 6 SERVINGS

PREP TIME 10 MINUTES

COOK TIME 30 MINUTES

EGG FREE, low LOW FODMAP, NUT FREE

(IF YOU DON'T NEED LOW FODMAP, YOU MAY USE WHITE ONION IN PLACE OF THE GREEN ONION AND 3 GARLIC CLOVES, CHOPPED, IN PLACE OF THE GARLIC-INFUSED OLIVE OIL.)

4 cups (364 g) chopped broccoli

2 cups (300 g) chopped carrots (about 3 medium carrots)

1½ pounds (680 g) potatoes, chopped

7 cups (1.7 L) water

1 teaspoon salt

2 tablespoons (30 ml) garlic-infused olive oil

¼ cup (24 g) chopped green onion

2 tablespoons (30 ml) lemon juice

1 cup (240 ml) full-fat coconut milk

1 teaspoon turmeric

There is no cheese in this soup, but you won't even be able to tell. The carrots give it the classic look and the lemon juice gives it tang. It's thick, creamy, and loaded with broccoli.

1. Combine the broccoli, carrots, potatoes, water, salt, olive oil, and green onion in a large stockpot and bring to a boil over high heat.

2. Decrease the heat to medium, cover, and cook for 15–20 minutes, or until the carrots are tender. Remove from the heat. Add the lemon juice, coconut milk, and turmeric.

3. Blend the soup completely with an immersion blender. Alternatively, transfer batches to a high-powered blender and blend. Be sure to remove the top piece of the lid of the blender and cover with a kitchen towel. This will let the heat release safely.

4. Ladle into bowls and serve immediately.

5. Store leftovers, covered, in the refrigerator for up to a week.

stuffed pepper soup

YIELD 8-10 SERVINGS

PREP TIME 15 MINUTES

COOK TIME 15 MINUTES

EGG FREE, **low** LOW FODMAP,
NUT FREE

This is way less work than stuffed peppers, but has all the same goodness. This is a hearty and easy soup that has been my go-to for years because it comes together quickly and is a crowd-pleaser. I have made it for birthday parties and family gatherings, and it always disappears quickly.

2 tablespoons (30 ml) garlic-infused olive oil

2 pounds (907 g) grass-fed ground beef

1 teaspoon salt

2 teaspoons (5 g) Italian seasoning

Two 14.5-ounce (411 g) cans fire-roasted diced tomatoes

1 cup (242 g) strained tomatoes (or tomato sauce, if low FODMAP isn't needed)

3 whole bell peppers (not green), cored and chopped

1 bunch green onions, chopped (about ½ cup [48 g])

3 cups (85 g) cooked cauliflower rice (optional) (not low FODMAP)

PRESSURE COOKER

1. Press Sauté on the pressure cooker. Add the olive oil, beef, salt, and seasoning and cook, breaking up the meat with a spoon and stirring regularly, for 6–8 minutes. Press Cancel.

2. Add the tomatoes, peppers, and green onions and stir well.

3. Place the lid on and make sure the valve is closed. Press Manual and then adjust the time to 10 minutes.

4. Press Cancel and release the pressure. Stir in the cauliflower rice, if desired. Serve hot.

STOVE

1. Heat the olive oil in a large skillet over medium heat. Add the peppers and cook, stirring, for 5 minutes, or until tender.

2. Add the beef, salt, and seasoning and cook for 5–7 minutes, or until the meat is browned.

3. Add the tomatoes, green onions, and ½ cup (120 ml) water and cook for 10 minutes. Add the cauliflower rice, if using. Serve hot.

sweet potato bacon chowder

YIELD 6-8 SERVINGS

PREP TIME 15 MINUTES

COOK TIME 20 MINUTES

EGG FREE, **low** LOW FODMAP,
NUT FREE IF COCONUT MILK IS USED
IN PLACE OF ALMOND MILK

(IF YOU DON'T NEED LOW FODMAP,
YOU MAY USE 1 TEASPOON GARLIC
POWDER IN PLACE OF THE
GARLIC-INFUSED OLIVE OIL.)

6 cups (870 g) peeled and chopped
sweet potatoes (about 3 medium
sweet potatoes)

5 cups (1.2 L) water

1 teaspoon salt

1 tablespoon (15 ml) garlic-infused
olive oil

1 teaspoon chopped fresh thyme

1 cup (240 ml) almond milk

3 cups (128 g) baby kale or spinach

12 ounces (340 g) bacon, cooked
and crumbled

This soup was born out of a need to use the sweet potatoes that I had bought too many of. Adding bacon is always a good option, for the crispiness and smokiness. The soup is creamy and thick. You can blend it fully for total creaminess or leave chunks of sweet potato; it's personal preference. You will love this simple yet satisfying soup.

1. Place the sweet potatoes, water, salt, olive oil, and thyme in a large stockpot. Bring to a boil over high heat, decrease the heat to medium-low, and cook for 15 minutes, or until the potatoes are tender.

2. Remove from the heat, add the almond milk, and blend with an immersion blender. Blend completely for a smooth soup or partially to leave chunks.

3. Add the kale and cook for 3–5 minutes, or until wilted.

4. Sprinkle the bacon on top when serving, so it doesn't get soggy.

5. Store leftovers, covered, in the refrigerator for up to a week.

Recipes

Chapter 9

desserts

Baking with grain-free flours is different from baking with traditional ingredients, but it can result in treats that are just as tasty. Living a paleo lifestyle does not mean you can never enjoy your favorite treat again—it just means you have to find a new way to make it. This chapter was my favorite to work on, and I know you will find recipes that you will love. I tested and retested multiple times to get them perfect so you have success the first time. If you have had paleo baking fails in the past, I encourage you to try one of these; I think it will be a success. Whether it's muffins, cakes, cookies, or brownies, you're sure to find a new favorite.

sweet potato brownies

YIELD 12 BROWNIES

PREP TIME 10 MINUTES

COOK TIME 18 MINUTES

The sweet potato is undetectable in these brownies, but it adds moisture and helps keep them fudgy.

¾ cup (172 g) mashed cooked sweet potato

½ cup (120 g) almond butter

½ cup (96 g) coconut sugar

2 large eggs

⅓ cup (27 g) cacao powder

½ cup (56 g) almond flour

2 tablespoons (15 g) coconut flour

¼ teaspoon salt

½ teaspoon ground cinnamon

¼ cup (45 g) dairy-free chocolate chips

1. Preheat the oven to 350°F (180°C or gas mark 4). Line a 9 by 9-inch (23 by 23 cm) pan with parchment paper or grease well with coconut oil.

2. Combine the sweet potato, almond butter, coconut sugar, and eggs in a large bowl. Mix with a hand mixer until well combined.

3. Add the cacao powder, almond flour, coconut flour, salt, and cinnamon. Mix with the hand mixer until fully combined. Add the chocolate chips and stir by hand.

4. Scoop into the prepared pan, spread evenly, and bake for 18 minutes, or until set.

5. Let cool, and then cut and serve.

6. Store leftovers, covered, in the refrigerator for up to 10 days.

pecan brownies

YIELD 12 BROWNIES

PREP TIME 10 MINUTES

COOK TIME 30 MINUTES

EGG FREE IF CHIA EGGS ARE USED

BROWNIES

¼ cup (60 g) almond or pecan butter

¼ cup (48 g) coconut sugar

⅓ cup (80 ml) maple syrup

¼ cup (60 ml) melted refined coconut oil

2 large eggs

1 teaspoon vanilla extract

¼ teaspoon salt

½ cup (56 g) almond flour

¾ cup (75 g) cacao powder

⅓ cup (37 g) chopped pecans

¼ cup (45 g) dairy-free chocolate chips

TOPPING

½ cup (56 g) chopped pecans

1 tablespoon (15 ml) maple syrup

These brownies are incredibly rich and feature buttery pecans. The combo is out-of-this-world good!

1. Preheat the oven to 325°F (170°C or gas mark 3). Line a 9 by 9-inch (23 by 23 cm) pan with parchment paper.

2. Make the brownies: Combine the almond butter, coconut sugar, maple syrup, coconut oil, eggs, and vanilla in a large bowl. Stir until smooth. Add the salt and almond flour and mix to combine. Add the pecans and chocolate chips and stir well. Scoop the mixture into the prepared pan and spread evenly.

3. Make the topping: Combine the pecans and maple syrup in a small bowl. Spread them on top of the brownies, pressing in lightly to help them stick.

4. Bake for 30 minutes, or until set. Let cool, and then cut and serve. These are very fudgy, so if you cut right away, they will be messy.

5. Store leftovers, covered, in the refrigerator for up to 10 days.

Tip: To substitute chia eggs: Mix 2 tablespoons (14 g) chia seeds with 5 tablespoons (75 ml) water and let sit for 5 minutes to thicken.

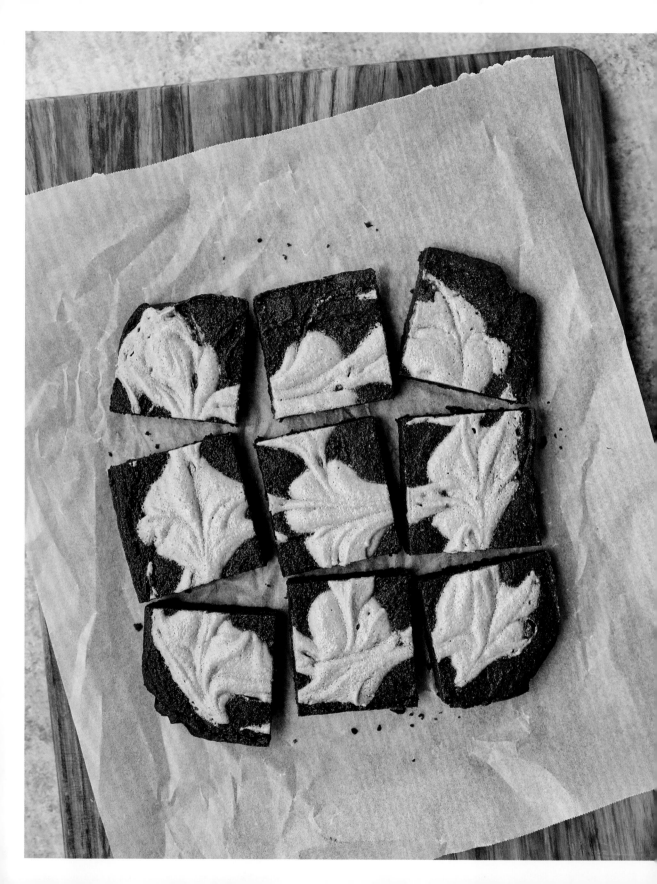

cashew butter swirl brownies

YIELD 12 BROWNIES

PREP TIME 10 MINUTES

COOK TIME 20 MINUTES

These brownies are super fudgy and have a sweet swirl of cashew butter on top. They are pretty, but they taste even better than they look.

BROWNIES

⅔ cup (128 g) coconut sugar

½ cup (120 ml) melted butter-flavored coconut oil

3 large eggs, at room temperature

1 teaspoon vanilla extract

½ cup (56 g) almond flour

⅓ cup (27 g) cacao powder

2 tablespoons (15 g) coconut flour

¼ teaspoon salt

2 tablespoons (30 ml) water

CASHEW BUTTER SWIRL

½ cup (120 g) cashew butter

2 tablespoons (30 ml) maple syrup

1 tablespoon (15 ml) melted coconut oil

1. Preheat the oven to 350°F (180°C or gas mark 4). Line a 9 by 9-inch (23 by 23 cm) baking pan with parchment paper.

2. Make the brownies: Combine the coconut sugar, coconut oil, eggs, and vanilla in a large bowl. Stir until well combined. Add the almond flour, cacao powder, coconut flour, salt, and water and stir until no dry spots remain. Scoop into the prepared pan and spread evenly.

3. Make the swirl: Combine the cashew butter, maple syrup, and coconut oil in a small bowl. Stir until smooth. Drop spoonfuls of the mixture on top of the brownies and use a butter knife to swirl the cashew butter with the brownie mixture. Swirl the knife back and forth or in circles.

4. Bake for 20 minutes, or until set.

5. Let cool, and then cut and serve.

6. Store leftovers, covered, in the refrigerator for up to a week.

strawberry mini cheesecakes

YIELD 10 SERVINGS

PREP TIME 20 MINUTES

CHILL TIME AT LEAST 2 HOURS

EGG FREE

CRUST

1 cup (116 g) raw almonds

1 cup (135 g) pitted dates

¼ teaspoon salt

1 tablespoon (15 ml) lemon juice

CHEESECAKE

2 cups (290 g) raw cashews, soaked in water for at least 4 hours

¼ cup (60 ml) melted coconut oil

3 tablespoons (45 ml) maple syrup

1 tablespoon (15 ml) lemon juice

½ teaspoon salt

1 teaspoon vanilla extract

8 ounces (227 g) strawberries, stemmed and sliced

Cheesecake with no dairy is possible. The lemon juice gives it the tang that usually comes from the cream cheese. This dessert is no-bake, not too sweet, and so heavenly. You'll need to soak the cashews for 4 hours ahead of time, but if you are in a hurry, soak the cashews in hot water for 1 hour; change the water a couple times as it cools.

1. Line a muffin tin with 10 parchment liners.

2. Make the crust: Place the almonds, dates, salt, and lemon juice in a food processor or high-powered blender. Process until the mixture is combined. It should stick together easily and the almonds should be broken down.

3. Divide the mixture among the 10 muffin liners and press down into crusts. Place in the refrigerator while you make the cheesecake.

4. Make the cheesecake: Drain the cashews and rinse with water. Place the cashews in a high-powdered blender. Add the coconut oil, maple syrup, lemon juice, salt, and vanilla. Blend on high speed until smooth. Add the strawberries and blend again until no pieces remain.

5. Remove the muffin tin from the refrigerator and pour the cheesecake filling on top of each crust. Place in the refrigerator for at least 2 hours to chill, or in the freezer for firmer cheesecakes.

6. Once firm, remove the cheesecakes from the tin and serve.

7. Store leftovers, covered, in the refrigerator for up to 10 days or freeze for up to 3 months.

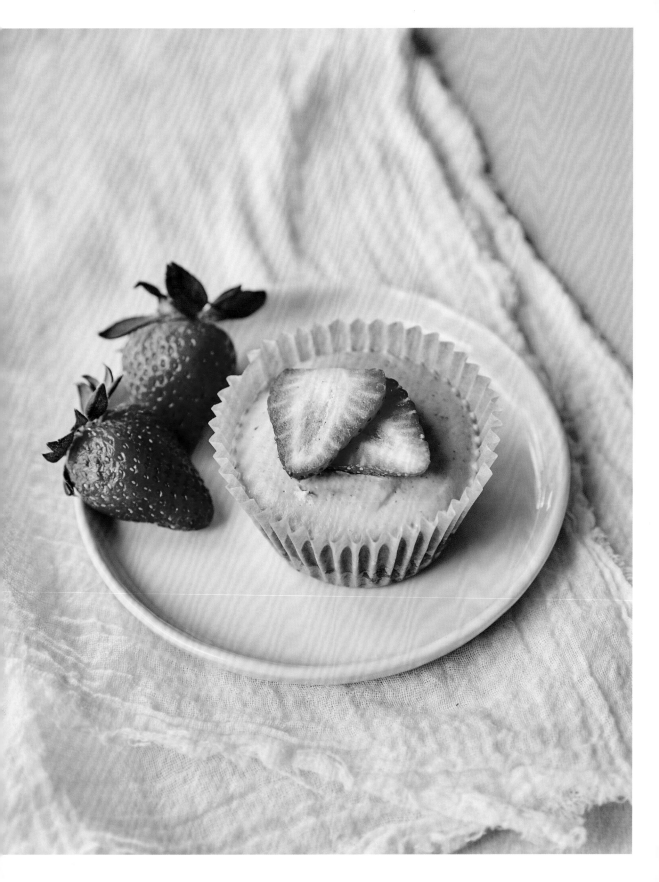

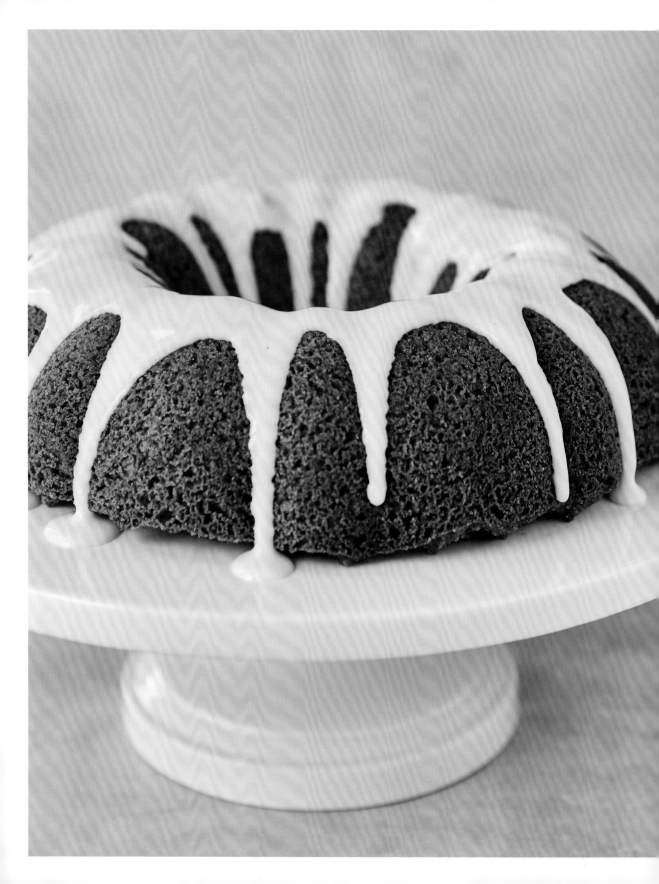

lemon poppy seed bundt cake

YIELD 8-10 SERVINGS

PREP TIME 10 MINUTES

COOK TIME 45 MINUTES

This cake is moist, tender, and sweet. Topped with a simple and bright glaze, it is fancy enough for a special occasion and easy enough to whip up anytime.

CAKE

3 cups (336 g) almond flour

⅓ cup (40 g) coconut flour

3 tablespoons (29 g) poppy seeds

2 teaspoons (10 g) baking soda

¾ teaspoon salt

½ cup (120 g) ghee

⅔ cup (128 g) coconut sugar

3 large eggs, at room temperature

Zest of 2 lemons

½ cup (120 ml) lemon juice (from 3 lemons)

¼ cup (60 ml) water

GLAZE

¼ cup (60 g) coconut butter/manna

1 tablespoon (15 ml) maple syrup

2 tablespoons (30 ml) lemon juice

⅛ teaspoon salt

1 teaspoon vanilla extract

1. Preheat the oven to 325°F (170°C or gas mark 3). Grease a 12-cup (3 L) Bundt pan very well with coconut oil or ghee.

2. Make the cake: Combine the almond flour, coconut flour, poppy seeds, baking soda, and salt in a medium-size bowl.

3. Combine the ghee and coconut sugar in a large bowl. Cream with a hand mixer. Add the eggs and mix again until smooth. Add the lemon zest, juice, and water and mix again.

4. Add in the dry mixture and mix well, until no dry spots remain.

5. Pour into the prepared pan and bake for 45 minutes, or until set. Let cool for 30 minutes and then remove from the pan. I always have good luck carefully loosening it first with a butter knife along the sides. Place a large plate on top of the pan and flip it over to release the cake.

6. Make the glaze: If the coconut butter is very hard, place it in the microwave for 30 seconds and stir well to combine. Combine the coconut butter, maple syrup, lemon juice, salt, and vanilla in a small bowl. Mix well and drizzle on top of the cake. Slice and serve.

7. Store leftovers, covered, at room temperature for 2 days, or refrigerated for longer.

orange cinnamon roll coffee cake

YIELD 9 SERVINGS

PREP TIME 20 MINUTES

COOK TIME 45 MINUTES

My dad always used to make orange cinnamon rolls from a can on weekend mornings. They weren't healthy, but I loved them. The sweet orange and cinnamon glaze of this dessert is inspired by those rolls, but it's made with real food ingredients.

CINNAMON-SUGAR MIXTURE

¼ cup (48 g) coconut sugar

2 teaspoons (5 g) ground cinnamon

COFFEE CAKE

3 cups (336 g) almond flour

¼ cup (30 g) coconut flour

1 teaspoon baking soda

½ teaspoon salt

½ cup (104 g) plus 1 tablespoon (13 g) coconut oil, at room temperature, divided

¾ cup (144 g) coconut sugar

3 eggs, at room temperature

1 teaspoon vanilla extract

Zest of 1 orange

½ cup (120 ml) orange juice (from 2 oranges)

2 tablespoons (30 ml) water

GLAZE

¼ cup (60 g) coconut butter

2 tablespoons (30 ml) maple syrup

3 tablespoons (45 ml) orange juice

1. Make the cinnamon-sugar mixture: Combine the coconut sugar and cinnamon in a small bowl. Mix well and set aside.

2. Make the coffee cake: Preheat the oven to 325°F (170°C or gas mark 3). Line a 9 by 9-inch (23 by 23 cm) pan with parchment paper.

3. Combine the almond flour, coconut flour, baking soda, and salt in a medium-size bowl. Stir until evenly mixed.

4. Place ½ cup (104 g) of the coconut oil and the coconut sugar in a large bowl and mix until combined. Add the eggs, vanilla, orange zest, orange juice, and water and stir until smooth.

5. Add the dry ingredients to the wet ingredients and stir well, making sure no dry spots remain.

6. Pour half of the batter into the prepared pan and sprinkle two-thirds of the cinnamon-sugar mixture on top. Carefully scoop the remaining batter on top, making sure all the cinnamon-sugar mixture is covered.

7. Bake for 45 minutes, or until set.

8. As soon as the cake comes out of the oven, spread the remaining 1 tablespoon (13 g) coconut oil on top and sprinkle with the remaining one-third cinnamon-sugar mixture.

9. While the cake is cooling, make the glaze: Combine the coconut butter, maple syrup, and orange juice in a small bowl. Mix until smooth and thin enough to drizzle on the cake.

10. Once the cake has cooled, top with the glaze. You can top it while it's warm, but it won't be as pretty. Slice and serve.

11. Store leftovers, covered, in the refrigerator for up to a week.

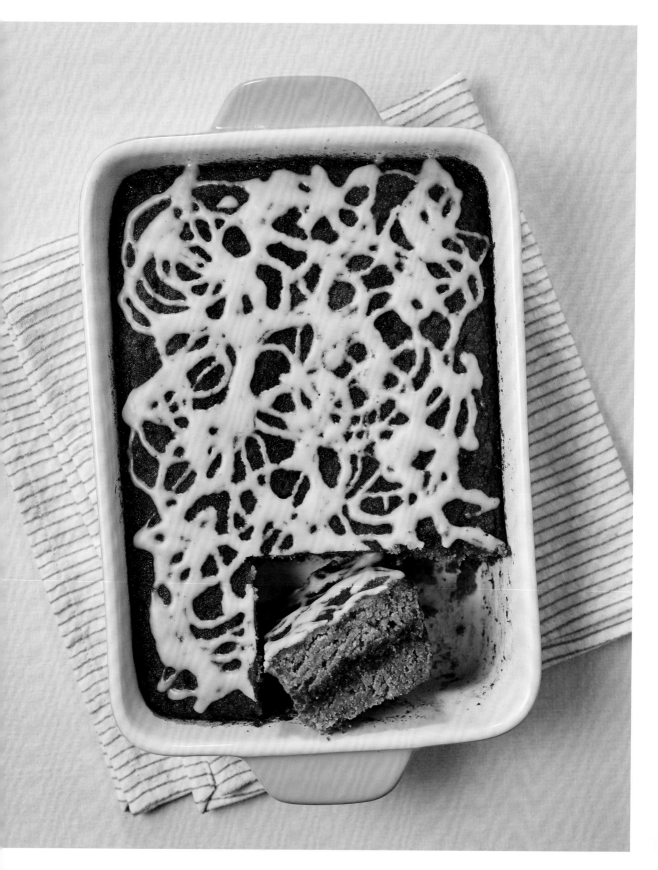

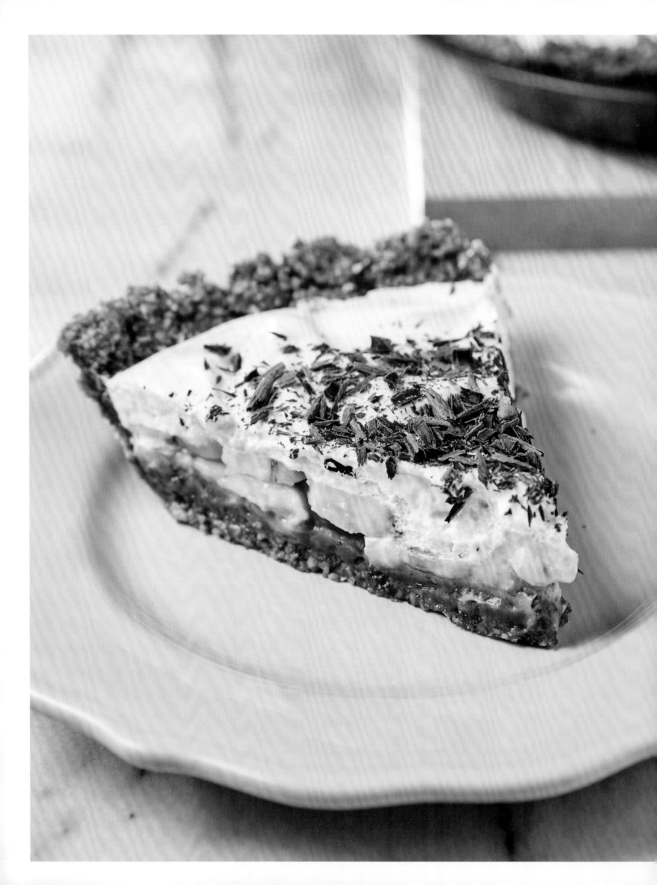

banoffee pie

YIELD 6-8 SERVINGS

PREP TIME 30 MINUTES

COOK TIME N/A

NUT FREE

(IF YOU DON'T NEED NUT FREE, USE
ANY NUT FOR THE CRUST AND ANY
NUT BUTTER FOR THE CARAMEL.)

CRUST

2 cups (299 g) raw sunflower seeds

1 cup (135 g) pitted dates

¼ teaspoon salt

2-3 tablespoons (30-45 ml) water

CARAMEL

1 cup (135 g) pitted dates

½ cup (128 g) sunflower seed butter,
such as SunButter

¼ teaspoon salt

2 teaspoons (10 ml) vanilla extract

3-4 tablespoons (45-60 ml) water

PIE

3 bananas, sliced into ¼-inch (6 mm)
slices

1-2 tablespoons (15-30 ml) lemon
juice

9 ounces (255 g) coconut whipped
topping

1 ounce (28 g) dairy-free chocolate,
shaved (optional)

*This banana toffee pie is incredibly rich. It's a no-bake dessert
that has a sweet caramel layer topped with thick banana slices
and a mountain of billowy coconut whipped cream.*

1. Line a deep-dish pie pan with parchment paper.

2. Make the crust: Combine the sunflower seeds, dates, and salt
   in a food processor and blend until mostly combined. Add
   the water, starting with 2 tablespoons (30 ml) and adding the
   rest if needed. The mixture should hold together, but it will be
   sticky. Press into the bottom and up the sides of the pie plate.
   Place in the refrigerator while you make the caramel.

3. Make the caramel: Combine the dates, sunflower seed butter,
   salt, and vanilla in a food processor. Add the water, starting
   with 3 tablespoons (45 ml) and adding the rest if needed, and
   blend until smooth. Scoop the mixture on top of the crust
   and smooth evenly. (If making ahead, stop at this step, cover,
   and refrigerate.)

4. Make the pie: Place the bananas in a medium-size bowl and
   add the lemon juice. Gently toss to cover all the banana slices.
   Evenly arrange the bananas on top of the caramel.

5. Top with the coconut whipped topping and serve immediately, or place in the refrigerator until serving. Dust with the
   shaved chocolate before serving, if desired.

6. This pie is best served the same day, but it can be stored,
   covered, in the refrigerator for up to 3 days.

banana blondies

YIELD 12 BLONDIES

PREP TIME 15 MINUTES

COOK TIME 40 MINUTES

EGG FREE

I love making banana bread, but sometimes I want a different treat with the ripe bananas needing to be used. These thick, moist bars are sweet and soft and taste similar to banana bread, but in bar form. The frosting makes them extra delicious.

BLONDIES

2 cups (224 g) almond flour

¼ cup (30 g) coconut flour

½ cup (96 g) coconut sugar

½ teaspoon salt

1½ teaspoons (4 g) ground cinnamon

½ cup (120 ml) almond milk

1 cup (240 ml) pureed banana
(2½–3 medium bananas)

FROSTING

¼ cup (62 g) coconut butter/manna

¼ cup (60 ml) maple syrup

⅛ teaspoon salt

1 teaspoon vanilla extract

2 tablespoons (26 g) butter-flavored coconut oil

1. Preheat the oven to 350°F (180°C or gas mark 4). Line a 9 by 9-inch (23 by 23 cm) pan with parchment paper or grease well with coconut oil.

2. Make the blondies: Combine the almond flour, coconut flour, coconut sugar, salt, and cinnamon in a large bowl and stir well. Add the almond milk and banana and mix until no dry spots remain. The mixture will be thick. Scoop into the prepared pan and bake for 35–40 minutes, or until set. Let cool before frosting.

3. Make the frosting: Combine the coconut butter, maple syrup, salt, vanilla, and coconut oil in a small bowl. Stir until well mixed and smooth. Spread over the blondies and place in the refrigerator to chill.

4. Slice and serve.

5. Store leftovers, covered, in the refrigerator for up to a week.

citrus snack cake

YIELD 8 SERVINGS

PREP TIME 15 MINUTES

COOK TIME 35 MINUTES

3 cups (336 g) almond flour

¾ cup (108 g) maple sugar or (144 g) coconut sugar

¼ cup (30 g) coconut flour

1 teaspoon baking soda

¼ teaspoon salt

Zest of 1 orange

Zest of 1 lemon

3 large eggs, at room temperature

½ cup (120 ml) melted ghee or butter-flavored coconut oil

¼ cup (60 ml) lemon juice

¼ cup (60 ml) orange juice

1 teaspoon vanilla extract

The combination of orange and lemon in this cake is wonderfully refreshing. It is simple to make and moist—a nice, light treat.

1. Preheat the oven to 325°F (170°C or gas mark 3). Line a 9-inch (23 cm) round pan with parchment paper or grease well with coconut oil.

2. Combine the almond flour, maple sugar, coconut flour, baking soda, and salt in a large bowl. Mix well.

3. Add the orange and lemon zests, eggs, ghee, lemon and orange juices, and vanilla. Stir well, until everything is mixed and no dry spots remain.

4. Pour into the prepared pan and bake for 35 minutes, or until set.

5. Let cool, then slice and serve warm. This is also great cold from the fridge.

6. Store leftovers, covered, in the refrigerator for up to a week.

butternut squash pecan crumble

YIELD 6 SERVINGS

PREP TIME 15 MINUTES

COOK TIME 1 HOUR 25 MINUTES

low LOW FODMAP

I don't tolerate pumpkin well, but I wanted a pumpkin-like dessert and this turned out better than I planned. It's a smooth, creamy layer of squash topped with the best-ever crumb topping. I served this at my family Thanksgiving and it was a huge hit. It will definitely become a yearly tradition.

SQUASH FILLING

1 butternut squash (about 3½ pounds [1.6 kg])

2 tablespoons (30 g) ghee

2 tablespoons (30 ml) maple syrup

2 large eggs

½ teaspoon salt

1 teaspoon ground cinnamon

1 teaspoon pumpkin pie spice

¼ cup (30 g) coconut flour

TOPPING

1½ cups (168 g) finely chopped raw pecans

¼ cup (30 g) coconut flour

3 tablespoons (40 g) ghee, at room temperature

1 teaspoon ground cinnamon

2 tablespoons (30 ml) maple syrup

¼ teaspoon salt

1. Preheat the oven to 425°F (220°C or gas mark 7). Line a baking sheet with parchment paper. Line a 9 by 9-inch (23 by 23 cm) pan with parchment paper or grease well with coconut oil.

2. Make the squash filling: Cut the butternut squash lengthwise and scoop out the seeds. Place cut side down on the prepared baking sheet and bake for 50–55 minutes, or until tender. Let cool for about 15 minutes, or until easily handled but still warm. Decrease the heat to 350°F (180°C or gas mark 4).

3. Scoop the squash into a large bowl. Add the ghee, maple syrup, eggs, salt, cinnamon, pumpkin pie spice, and coconut flour. Stir well, mashing any chunks. Use an immersion blender if you want it really smooth.

4. Scoop the butternut squash mixture into the prepared pan.

5. Make the topping: Combine the pecans, coconut flour, ghee, cinnamon, maple syrup, and salt in a medium-size bowl. Mix until combined and crumbly. Evenly sprinkle the mixture on top of the squash.

6. Bake for 30 minutes, or until the top is lightly brown.

7. Let cool, then slice and serve.

8. Store leftovers, covered, in the refrigerator for up to a week.

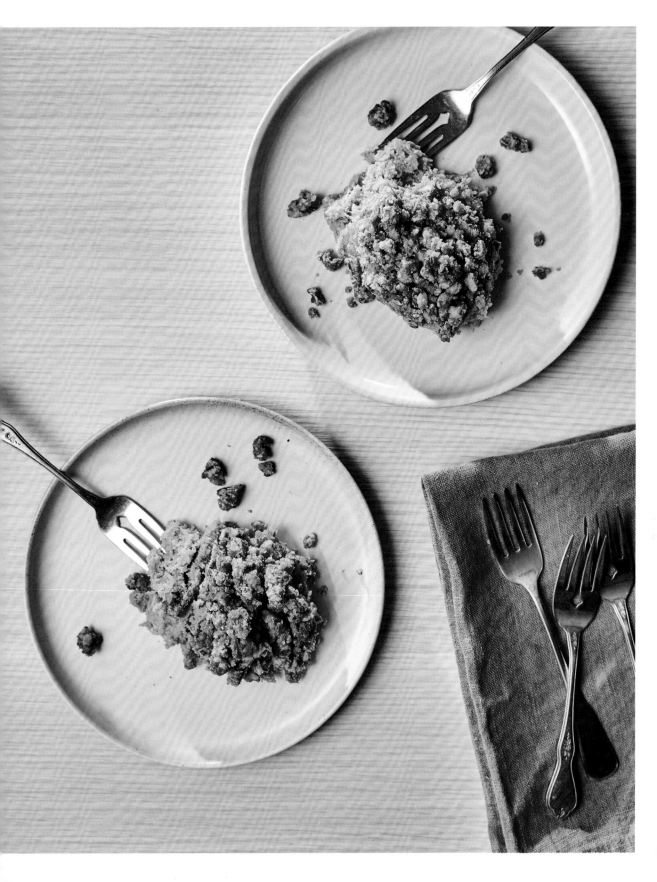

german chocolate ice cream

YIELD 6–8 SERVINGS

PREP TIME 10 MINUTES

COOK TIME 10 MINUTES,
PLUS 2 HOURS OF CHILLING

EGG FREE

ICE CREAM

Two 13.5-ounce (378 ml) cans full-fat coconut milk

⅓ cup (80 ml) maple syrup

¼ cup (45 g) dairy-free chocolate chips

¼ cup (20 g) cacao powder

¼ cup (60 g) almond butter

¼ teaspoon salt

COCONUT-PECAN MIXTURE

¾ cup (70 g) finely shredded unsweetened coconut

1 cup (135 g) pitted dates

2 tablespoons (30 g) almond butter

1 teaspoon (5 ml) vanilla extract

3 tablespoons (45 ml) warm water

¼ teaspoon salt

1 cup (112 g) roughly chopped pecans

Homemade ice cream may sound like a complicated dessert, but it's really one of the easiest treats to make. The ice cream base is combined over the stove and then chilled and the coconut mixture is made in the blender. They come together to make a rich and decadent dessert that you will love. It is a creamy chocolate ice cream studded with chunks of a divine coconut–pecan mixture.

1. Before you begin, freeze an ice cream bowl for at least 24 hours.

2. Make the ice cream mixture: Add the coconut milk, maple syrup, chocolate chips, cacao powder, almond butter, and salt to a 2-quart (2 L) saucepan over medium heat and whisk for 3–5 minutes, or until the mixture is smooth and the chocolate has fully melted. Remove from the heat and pour into a glass bowl. Let cool. Cover and refrigerate for at least 2 hours or overnight.

3. Make the coconut-pecan mixture: Preheat the oven to 350°F (180°C or gas mark 4). Line a baking sheet with parchment paper. Line a loaf pan with parchment paper.

4. Spread the coconut on the prepared baking sheet. Bake for 5 minutes, or until lightly golden brown.

5. Combine the toasted coconut, dates, almond butter, vanilla, water, and salt in a food processor or high-powdered blender. Blend until combined. It will be thick, like dough.

6. Pour the cooled ice cream mixture into your ice cream maker and follow the manufacturer's instructions for churning. Mine took 6–8 minutes. Add the chopped pecans during the last 1–2 minutes. Scoop into the prepared loaf pan, a little at a time, while adding dollops of the coconut mixture. Continue until all the ice cream and coconut mixture is in the pan. Spread evenly and place in the freezer for at least 4 hours.

7. Scoop and serve.

blueberry cheesecake ice cream

YIELD 6-8 SERVINGS

PREP TIME 15 MINUTES

COOK TIME 6 MINUTES, PLUS 2 HOURS OF CHILLING

EGG FREE, NUT FREE

Two 13.5-ounce (378 ml) cans full-fat coconut milk

¼ cup (60 ml) maple syrup

2 teaspoons (12 g) grass-fed gelatin

¾ cup (180 g) cashew butter

2 tablespoons (30 ml) lemon juice

1 teaspoon vanilla extract

1½ cups (222 g) fresh or (233 g) frozen blueberries

This creamy, rich ice cream is studded with juicy blueberries. The cashew butter and lemon juice mixture gives it a cheesecake flavor without the dairy.

1. Before you begin, freeze an ice cream bowl for at least 24 hours.

2. Whisk the coconut milk and maple syrup in a 2-quart (2 L) saucepan. Sprinkle the gelatin on top and let bloom (just let it sit) for 5 minutes.

3. Combine the cashew butter and lemon juice in a small bowl.

4. Place the coconut milk mixture over medium heat and cook for about 3 minutes, or until thick with no remaining lumps. Stir in the cashew butter mixture and whisk for 2–3 minutes, or until combined. Turn off the heat and add the vanilla.

5. Pour the mixture into a glass container. Let cool. Cover and place in the refrigerator for at least 2 hours or overnight.

6. Once the mixture is chilled, pour into an ice cream maker and churn according to the manufacturer's instructions. It took mine 10 minutes. Add the blueberries during the last 2 minutes.

7. While the ice cream is churning, prepare a loaf pan by lining it with parchment paper.

8. Scoop the ice cream into the prepared loaf pan and place in the freezer, or serve immediately for soft-serve consistency.

peppermint patties

YIELD 16 PATTIES

PREP TIME 20 MINUTES, PLUS 2 HOURS OF CHILLING

COOK TIME N/A

EGG FREE, NUT FREE

What's better than a creamy cool peppermint center encased by sweet dark chocolate? One that's simple to make. These also make a great gift, because they don't need to be kept in the refrigerator.

¾ cup (186 g) coconut butter/manna

¼ cup (60 ml) melted coconut oil

3–4 tablespoons (45–60 ml) maple syrup

⅛ teaspoon salt

1½ teaspoons (7 ml) peppermint extract

1 cup (180 g) dairy-free chocolate chips

1. Make sure the coconut butter is soft. If it's hard, warm briefly in the microwave and stir well. Line a baking sheet with parchment or wax paper.

2. Combine the coconut butter, coconut oil, maple syrup, salt, and peppermint extract in a small bowl. Mix well. Refrigerate for 10 minutes to firm up.

3. Roll into 1½-teaspoon balls and press into 1½-inch (4 cm) circles, forming patties. Place on the prepared baking sheet. Repeat with the remaining mixture; it should make 16 total.

4. Place in the refrigerator for 2 hours to chill.

5. Melt the chocolate chips in the microwave, stirring every 30 seconds, for about 1½ minutes, or until smooth. Alternatively, melt the chocolate in a small saucepan over low heat, stirring the whole time.

6. Dip the patties in the melted chocolate, letting the excess drip off, and place back on the baking sheet. Dip all of them and then place in the refrigerator to set.

7. Once set, they do not need to be refrigerated. Store leftovers, covered, at room temperature for up to a week.

chocolate cobbler

YIELD 6 SERVINGS

PREP TIME 10 MINUTES

COOK TIME 38 MINUTES

EGG FREE

CAKE

1½ cups (168 g) almond flour

2 tablespoons (15 g) coconut flour

¼ cup (20 g) cacao powder

⅓ cup (64 g) coconut sugar

¼ teaspoon salt

1 teaspoon baking soda

¼ cup (60 ml) melted ghee

½ cup (120 ml) almond milk

TOPPING

1 tablespoon (12 g) coconut sugar

1 tablespoon (5 g) cacao powder

¾ cup (180 ml) hot water

This cobbler is a cross between chocolate cake and pudding. It's moist, rich, and totally scrumptious.

1. Preheat the oven to 350°F (180°C or gas mark 4). Line a 9 by 9-inch (23 by 23 cm) pan with parchment or grease well with coconut oil.

2. Make the cake: Combine the almond flour, coconut flour, cacao powder, coconut sugar, salt, and baking soda in a large bowl. Stir well. Add the ghee and almond milk and stir. The mixture will be thick. Spread into the prepared pan.

3. Make the topping: Combine the coconut sugar and cacao powder in a small dish and sprinkle over the cake.

4. Pour the hot water evenly on top, don't mix, and bake for 35–38 minutes. Serve warm.

5. Store leftovers, covered, in the refrigerator for up to a week.

hot cocoa

YIELD 2 SERVINGS

PREP TIME 3 MINUTES

COOK TIME 3 MINUTES

EGG FREE, **low** LOW FODMAP,
NUT FREE IF COCONUT MILK IS
USED IN PLACE OF ALMOND MILK

1 cup (240 ml) almond milk

1 cup (240 ml) water

¼ cup (20 g) cacao powder

2 tablespoons (30 ml) maple syrup,
or to taste

There is something so nostalgic about a cup of creamy, sweet, and rich hot cocoa, the perfect treat on a cold day. This will be your go-to when you're craving a cup of something warm. This recipe can easily be doubled or tripled to serve more people.

1. Combine the almond milk, water, cacao powder, and maple syrup in a 2-quart (2 L) saucepan over medium heat. Whisk for 2–3 minutes, or until combined and warmed.

2. Serve warm.

3. Store any leftovers in a jar in the refrigerator, and shake before serving.

cinnamon roll scones

YIELD 6 SCONES

PREP TIME 10 MINUTES

COOK TIME 22 MINUTES

Tender scones, swirled with cinnamon sugar and drizzled with a sweet glaze, are great for breakfast or dessert.

SCONES

2 cups (224 g) almond flour

2 tablespoons (15 g) coconut flour

¼ cup (36 g) maple sugar or (38 g) coconut sugar

½ teaspoon salt

1 teaspoon baking soda

¼ cup (60 ml) melted ghee

1 large egg, at room temperature

2 tablespoons (30 ml) almond milk

1 teaspoon vanilla extract

CINNAMON-SUGAR TOPPING

2 tablespoons (18 g) maple sugar or (18 g) coconut sugar

2 teaspoons (5 g) ground cinnamon

GLAZE

¼ cup (60 g) coconut butter

2 tablespoons (30 ml) maple syrup

1 teaspoon vanilla

2 to 3 tablespoons (30 to 45 ml) water

1. Preheat the oven to 325°F (170°C or gas mark 3). Line a baking sheet with parchment paper.

2. Make the scones: Combine the almond flour, coconut flour, maple sugar, salt, and baking soda in a large bowl. Stir well.

3. Add the ghee, egg, almond milk, and vanilla. Stir until a dough is formed and no dry spots remain.

4. Make the cinnamon-sugar topping: Combine the maple sugar and cinnamon in a small bowl. Add half to the dough and mix slightly, leaving it with streaks. Reserve the remaining half for the top.

5. Press the dough into an 8-inch (20 cm) circle on the prepared baking sheet. Cut into 6 triangles by cutting in half and then cutting each half into thirds. Gently separate the scones, sprinkle the tops with the remaining cinnamon-sugar mixture, and bake for 20–22 minutes. These are best served fresh out of the oven.

6. Make the glaze: First make sure the coconut butter is smooth and creamy. If it's hard, heat it in the microwave for 30 seconds and then stir well. Combine coconut butter, maple syrup, vanilla, and water and stir until smooth. Drizzle over the scones.

7. Store leftovers, covered, in the refrigerator for up to a week. These also freeze well in an airtight bag.

pumpkin spice latte

YIELD 1–2 SERVINGS

PREP TIME 5 MINUTES

COOK TIME 4 MINUTES

EGG FREE, NUT FREE

This healthier, homemade version of the popular autumn drink is made with just a few simple ingredients and is ready in 10 minutes.

1 cup (240 ml) brewed coffee

¾ cup (180 ml) full-fat coconut milk

2 tablespoons (30 ml) maple syrup

2 tablespoons (34 g) canned pumpkin

½ teaspoon pumpkin pie spice

1. Combine the coffee, coconut milk, maple syrup, pumpkin, and pumpkin pie spice in a 2-quart (2 L) saucepan over medium heat. Whisk for 3–4 minutes, or until smooth and warmed.

2. Serve immediately.

chocolate mint cookies

YIELD 12 COOKIES

PREP TIME 10 MINUTES

COOK TIME 12 MINUTES

1 cup (116 g) raw almonds

1 cup (135 g) pitted dates

2 tablespoons (30 g) almond butter

½ teaspoon salt

¼ cup (20 g) cacao powder

¼ teaspoon baking soda

1 large egg

½ teaspoon peppermint extract

These cookies are mixed completely in the food processor, so they come together quickly. They are slightly crisp on the outside and the inside is fudgy.

1. Preheat the oven to 350°F (180°C or gas mark 4). Line a baking sheet with parchment paper.

2. Blend the almonds in a food processor until fine like flour. Add the dates and almond butter, and blend until it forms a sticky dough. Add the salt, cacao powder, baking soda, and egg and blend again until combined. Add the peppermint extract and blend again.

3. Scoop into heaping tablespoon (15 g) portions, roll into balls, and place on the prepared baking sheet. Press down slightly and bake for 10–12 minutes. Serve warm, at room temperature, or chilled.

4. Store leftovers, covered, in the refrigerator for up to 10 days.

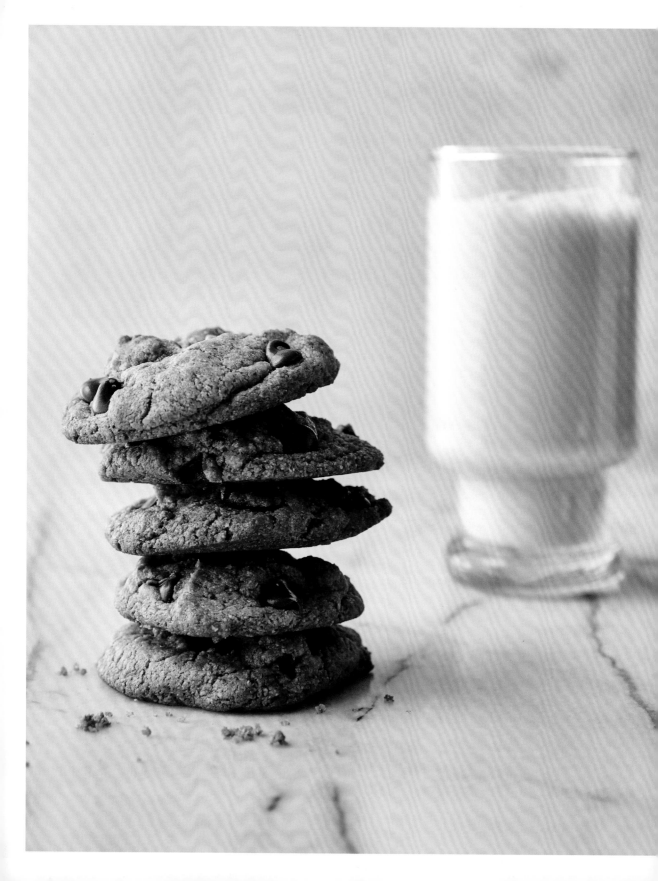

mike's favorite chocolate chip cookies

YIELD 18 COOKIES

PREP TIME 10 MINUTES

COOK TIME 12 MINUTES

6 tablespoons (90 g) ghee,
at room temperature

¾ cup (144 g) coconut sugar

1 large egg, at room temperature

⅓ cup (80 g) cashew butter

1¼ cups (140 g) almond flour

3 tablespoons (23 g) coconut flour

1 teaspoon vanilla extract

¼ teaspoon salt

1 teaspoon baking soda

1 cup (180 g) dairy-free chocolate
chips

Mike is a close family friend who helps me test recipes. These are his absolute favorite. At first he couldn't believe they were paleo, because they taste so much like the originals. If you are in search of the best chocolate chip cookie, this is it!

1. Preheat the oven to 350°F (180°C or gas mark 4). Line a baking sheet with parchment paper.

2. Combine the ghee and coconut sugar in a large bowl. Mix until well combined. A hand mixer works best for this. Add the egg and cashew butter and mix again until smooth. Add the almond flour, coconut flour, vanilla, salt, and baking soda and mix until no dry spots remain. Fold in the chocolate chips (keep some aside if you want to add more in step 3).

3. Scoop the mixture into heaping tablespoon (15 g) portions and roll into balls. Place them on the prepared baking sheet and press down just slightly. Add a couple more chocolate chips on top of each one, if desired.

4. Bake for 10–12 minutes, or until the edges look done. The center will still look soft. Let cool for at least 10 minutes before removing from the pan. They are soft when they first come out, but will firm up as they cool. They are great served warm.

5. Store leftovers, covered, at room temperature for up to 2 days or in the refrigerator for up to 10 days.

thick sugar cookies

YIELD 16 COOKIES

PREP TIME 10 MINUTES

COOK TIME 12 MINUTES

1⅔ cups (187 g) almond flour

3 tablespoons (23 g) coconut flour

½ teaspoon baking soda

¼ teaspoon salt

½ cup (120 g) ghee or (104 g) butter-flavored coconut oil, at room temperature

½ cup (72 g) maple sugar or (96 g) coconut sugar

1 large egg, at room temperature

1 teaspoon vanilla extract

These cookies are soft and sweet—the perfect cookies. They're an incredible remake of the classic that is so well loved. Maple sugar is lighter than coconut sugar, making cookies that look more like traditional sugar cookies. Coconut sugar works great as well, but the cookies will be slightly darker.

1. Preheat the oven to 325°F (170°C or gas mark 3). Line a baking sheet with parchment paper.

2. Combine the almond flour, coconut flour, baking soda, and salt in a medium-size bowl. Stir well.

3. Combine the ghee and maple sugar in a large bowl. Mix with a hand mixer until combined. Add the egg and vanilla and mix again until smooth.

4. Add the dry ingredients to the wet ingredients and mix again until fully combined, with no dry spots remaining.

5. Scoop into 1 tablespoon (15 g) portions, roll into balls, and place on the prepared baking sheet. Press down slightly and bake for 10–12 minutes. Serve warm or at room temperature.

6. Store leftovers, covered, in the refrigerator for up to 10 days.

maple pecan fudge

YIELD 8–10 SERVINGS

PREP TIME 10 MINUTES

COOK TIME N/A

EGG FREE

1 cup (240 g) cashew butter

¼ cup (60 ml) maple syrup

2 tablespoons (30 ml) melted coconut oil

1 teaspoon vanilla extract

2 tablespoons (15 g) coconut flour

⅓ cup (45 g) chopped pecans, divided

This combination of rich cashew butter, sweet maple syrup, and crunchy pecans is irresistible. It results in a melt-in-your-mouth fudge that everyone will love. It's a great no-bake treat to whip up and have on hand for when you need a little sweet bite.

1. Line a loaf pan with parchment paper.

2. Combine the cashew butter, maple syrup, coconut oil, and vanilla in a medium-size bowl. Stir well. Stir in the coconut flour until well combined. Add half the pecans. Scoop the mixture into the prepared pan and spread evenly.

3. Top with the remaining pecans, pressing them in slightly. Place in the refrigerator to set.

4. Slice and serve chilled.

5. Store leftovers, covered, in the refrigerator for up to 2 weeks.

classic chocolate fudge

YIELD 10–12 SERVINGS

PREP TIME 5 MINUTES

COOK TIME 45 MINUTES

EGG FREE, **low** LOW FODMAP, NUT FREE

One 13.5-ounce (378 ml) can full-fat coconut milk

⅓ cup (80 ml) maple syrup

⅛ teaspoon salt

2½ cups (450 g) unsweetened chocolate chips

1 teaspoon vanilla extract

This fudge makes a great gift, because it doesn't need to be kept in the refrigerator to stay firm. Making the homemade sweetened condensed milk takes a little time, but it's very easy. If you're looking for a fudge you can give or set out at parties, this is it!

1. Line a loaf pan with parchment paper or grease well with coconut oil.

2. Combine the coconut milk, maple syrup, and salt in a 2-quart (2 L) saucepan over medium heat and whisk until the mixture is boiling. Decrease the heat to low and simmer until the mixture is thickened, 25–45 minutes, depending on how low your setting goes. It should measure about 1¼ cups (300 ml) when done.

3. Place the chocolate chips in a large bowl. Pour the coconut milk mixture over the chocolate chips. The heat will melt them. Add the vanilla and stir until completely smooth.

4. Pour into the prepared pan and place in the refrigerator to set.

5. Once set, this does not need to be kept in the refrigerator. Slice and serve.

6. Store leftovers, covered, at room temperature for up to a week.

cheesecake dip

YIELD 2 CUPS (473 ML), ABOUT 10 SERVINGS

PREP TIME 10 MINUTES

COOK TIME N/A

EGG FREE

2 cups (300 g) raw cashews

3 tablespoons (45 ml) maple syrup

½ teaspoon salt

2 tablespoons (30 ml) lemon juice

1 teaspoon vanilla extract

Creamy and sweetened just right, this makes a great dip for fruit or grain-free cookies for an indulgent treat. You will need to soak the cashews for 6 hours. If you are short on time, soak them for 1 hour in hot water, changing the water a couple times as it cools.

1. Soak the cashews in water for 6 hours to soften. Drain, rinse the cashews, and place in a high-powdered blender.

2. Add the maple syrup, salt, lemon juice, and vanilla. Blend until smooth, stopping and scraping down the sides as needed. This may take 5–10 minutes; just be patient as you stop and scrape down. It will get smooth and creamy.

3. Pour into a serving bowl and serve immediately as a dip for fruit or grain-free cookies.

4. Store leftovers, covered, in the refrigerator for up to 10 days.

almond butter banana bundt cake

YIELD 8-10 SERVINGS

PREP TIME 15 MINUTES

COOK TIME 40 MINUTES

This is a soft and tender cake with a buttery crumb, topped with an incredible caramel-like glaze. It looks fancy but is easy to make.

CAKE

1 cup (225 g) mashed or pureed banana (about 3 medium bananas)

½ cup (96 g) coconut sugar

½ cup (120 g) almond butter

2 large eggs

1 teaspoon vanilla extract

3 cups (336 g) almond flour

¼ cup (30 g) coconut flour

1 teaspoon ground cinnamon

½ teaspoon salt

1 teaspoon baking soda

¾ cup (180 ml) almond milk

GLAZE

¼ cup (60 g) almond butter

¼ cup (60 ml) melted coconut oil

¼ cup (60 ml) maple syrup

1 teaspoon vanilla extract

1. Preheat the oven to 350°F (180°C or gas mark 4). Grease a 12-cup (3 L) Bundt pan well with coconut oil.

2. Make the cake: Combine the banana, coconut sugar, almond butter, eggs, and vanilla in a large bowl. Stir well.

3. In a separate bowl, add the almond flour, coconut flour, cinnamon, salt, and baking soda. Stir to combine. Add the dry ingredients to the wet and stir to combine. Add the almond milk and stir again until no dry spots remain.

4. Pour the mixture into the prepared Bundt pan and spread evenly. Bake for 40 minutes, or until set.

5. Let cool for 10 minutes. Remove from the pan. I always have good luck carefully loosening it first with a butter knife along the sides. Place a large plate on top and flip it over.

6. Make the glaze: Combine the almond butter, coconut oil, maple syrup, and vanilla in a small bowl. Stir until smooth. Drizzle over the cooled cake. Slice and serve.

7. Store leftovers, covered, in the refrigerator for up to a week.

pecan pie muffins

YIELD 9 MUFFINS

PREP TIME 10 MINUTES

COOK TIME 25 MINUTES

1 cup (112 g) almond flour

¾ cup (144 g) coconut sugar

¼ teaspoon salt

2 large eggs, at room temperature

⅓ cup (70 g) coconut oil, at room temperature

1 tablespoon (15 ml) molasses

1 cup (140 g) chopped raw pecans

½ cup (90 g) dairy-free chocolate chips (optional)

These are the most popular muffin recipe on my website, so I knew they needed to be included in this book! They are denser than a traditional muffin, way easier to make than pie, and incredibly delicious.

1. Preheat the oven to 325°F (170°C or gas mark 3). Line a muffin pan with 9 parchment liners.

2. Combine the almond flour, coconut sugar, and salt in a large bowl. Stir well.

3. Add the eggs, coconut oil, and molasses and stir well, until no dry spots remain. Stir in the pecans and chocolate chips, if using.

4. Scoop the batter into the muffin liners and bake for 25 minutes, or until the edges are slightly brown.

5. Let cool for 10 minutes, and then remove from the pan. Serve warm or at room temperature.

6. Store leftovers, covered, at room temperature for 3 days, or longer in the refrigerator.

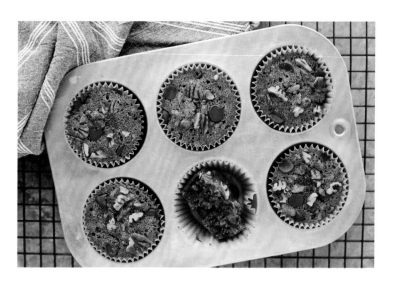

acknowledgments

——

To Sarah and Mike, thank you for being my official taste testers on all the recipes and offering feedback. I'm so glad I was able to share so many recipes with you both.

To Derek, thank you for your support and believing in me.

To my amazing publishing team, thank you for all the help along the way, leading and encouraging me through the whole process.

To Pat Mauk, who sparked my love of baking at a young age and forever changed my life.

And last, but certainly not least, my *Real Food with Jessica* community. Thank you to everyone who makes my recipes, reads my blog, comments, and supports me. This book is for you, and I couldn't have done it without you.

about the author

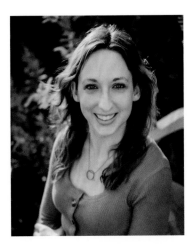

Jessica DeMay is a self-taught cook who began baking as a teenager and turned her passion into a full-time job and blog years later. She is known for her paleo desserts and family-friendly meals. She currently resides in Muskegon, Michigan, with her daughter, Joanna, who regularly helps her out in the kitchen. When they aren't baking, they are taking trips to the lake or crafting together. Besides being a mom, she spends her days running her food blog *Real Food with Jessica*. You can find more from her on her blog and Instagram @Realfoodwithjessica.

index